ICOG Campus
Male Infertility
Recent Developments and Current Practice

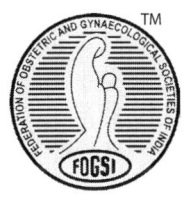 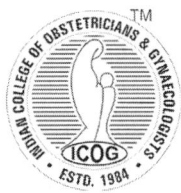

Indian College of Obstetricians & Gynaecologists

ICOG Campus

Male Infertility
Recent Developments and Current Practice

Jaydeep Tank
President, FOGSI

Parul J Kotdawala
Chairperson, ICOG

Madhuri Patel
Secretary General, FOGSI

Sarita Bhalerao
Secretary, ICOG

Editors

Pratik Tambe MD FICOG FICRM
ART Consultant and Gynec Endoscopic Surgeon
Department of Obstetrics and Gynecology
Ashirwad IVF
Mumbai, Maharashtra, India
Governing Council Member, ICOG (2020–2025)
Governing Council member, ICRM (2024–2026)
Chairperson, AMOGS Endocrinology Committee (2020–2024)
Chairperson, FOGSI Endocrinology Committee (2017–2019)
Managing Council Member, MOGS, ISAR, MSR

Asha R Rao MBBS MD (Obs & Gyne) FICOG
Infertility Specialist, Medical Director and Chief Consultant
Department of Obstetrics and Gynecology
Rao Hospital and Centre for Assisted Reproduction and Endoscopy (CARE)
Coimbatore, Tamil Nadu, India

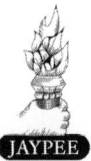

JAYPEE BROTHERS MEDICAL PUBLISHERS
The Health Sciences Publisher
New Delhi | London

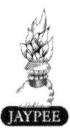 **Jaypee Brothers Medical Publishers (P) Ltd.**

Headquarters
Jaypee Brothers Medical Publishers (P) Ltd
EMCA House, 23/23-B
Ansari Road, Daryaganj
New Delhi 110 002, India
Landline: +91-11-23272143, +91-11-23272703
+91-11-23282021, +91-11-23245672
Email: jaypee@jaypeebrothers.com

Corporate Office
Jaypee Brothers Medical Publishers (P) Ltd
4838/24, Ansari Road, Daryaganj
New Delhi 110 002, India
Phone: +91-11-43574357
Fax: +91-11-43574314
Email: jaypee@jaypeebrothers.com

Overseas Office
JP Medical Ltd.
83, Victoria Street, London
SW1H 0HW (UK)
Phone: +44 20 3170 8910
Fax: +44 (0)20 3008 6180
Email: info@jpmedpub.com

Website: www.jaypeebrothers.com
Website: www.jaypeedigital.com

© 2024, Jaypee Brothers Medical Publishers

The views and opinions expressed in this book are solely those of the original contributor(s)/author(s) and do not necessarily represent those of editor(s) or publisher of the book.

All rights reserved. No part of this publication may be reproduced, stored or transmitted in any form or by any means, electronic, mechanical, photo copying, recording or otherwise, without the prior permission in writing of the publishers.

All brand names and product names used in this book are trade names, service marks, trademarks or registered trademarks of their respective owners. The publisher is not associated with any product or vendor mentioned in this book.

Medical knowledge and practice change constantly. This book is designed to provide accurate, authoritative information about the subject matter in question. However, readers are advised to check the most current information available on procedures included and check information from the manufacturer of each product to be administered, to verify the recommended dose, formula, method and duration of administration, adverse effects and contra indications. It is the responsibility of the practitioner to take all appropriate safety precautions. Neither the publisher nor the author(s)/editor(s) assume any liability for any injury and/or damage to persons or property arising from or related to use of material in this book.

This book is sold on the understanding that the publisher is not engaged in providing professional medical services. If such advice or services are required, the services of a competent medical professional should be sought.

Every effort has been made where necessary to contact holders of copyright to obtain permission to reproduce copyright material. If any have been inadvertently overlooked, the publisher will be pleased to make the necessary arrangements at the first opportunity.

Inquiries for bulk sales may be solicited at: jaypee@jaypeebrothers.com

ICOG Campus—Male Infertility: Recent Developments and Current Practice

First Edition: **2024**

ISBN: 978-93-5696-734-2

Printed in India

ICOG Office Bearers 2024

Dr Jaydeep Tank President, FOGSI	**Dr Parul J Kotdawala** Chairperson
Dr Sheela Mane Vice Chairperson	**Dr Sarita Bhalerao** Secretary
Dr Parag Biniwale Chairperson Elect	**Professor Ashok Kumar** Vice Chairperson Elect

ICOG Past Chairpersons

(Late) Dr CL Jhaveri Past Chairman (1989–1996) Mumbai	**(Late) Dr CS Dawn** Past Chairman (1997–1999) Kolkata	**(Late) Dr Behram Anklesaria** Past Chairman (2011) Ahmedabad
(Late) Dr Mahendra N Parikh Past Chairman (2000–2002)	**Dr Rohit V Bhatt** Past Chairman (2003–2005)	**Dr Usha B Saraiya** Past Chairman (2006–2008)
Dr Duru Shah Past Chairman (2009–2010)	**Dr AK Debdas** Past Chairman (2012)	**Dr Hiralal Konar** Past Chairman (2013)
Dr Atul Munshi Past Chairperson (2014)	**Dr Dilip Kumar Dutta** Past Chairperson (2015)	**Professor Krishnendu Gupta** Past Chairperson (2016)
Dr Mala Arora Past Chairperson (2017)	**Dr S Shantha Kumari** Past Chairperson (2018)	**Professor Tushar Kar** Past Chairperson (2019)
Dr Mandakini Megh Past Chairperson (2020–2021)	**Dr Uday Thanawala** Past Chairperson (2021–2022)	**Dr Laxmi Shrikhande** Imm Past Chairperson (Oct 2022–Dec 2023)

ICOG Governing Council Members (2024–2025)

Dr Achla Batra New Delhi	**Dr Anju Soni** Jaipur	**Dr Asha R Rao** Coimbatore
Dr Aswath Kumar Thrissur	**Dr Bharti Maheshwari** Meerut	**Dr Charmila A** Trichy
Dr Durga Shankar Dash Cuttack	**Dr Fessy Louis T** Kochi	**Dr Hafizur Rahman** Gangtok
Dr Haresh Doshi Ahmedabad	**Dr JB Sharma** New Delhi	**Dr Kavita N Singh** Jabalpur
Dr Kiran Pandey Kanpur	**Dr Komal Chavan** Mumbai	**Dr Meena Samant** Patna
Dr Pragya Mishra Patna	**Dr Pratik Tambe** Mumbai	**Dr Poonam Goyal** New Delhi
Dr Radhika AG New Delhi	**Dr Rakhi Singh** Noida	**Dr Ranjana Khanna** Allahabad
Dr Seema Pandey Azamgarh	**Dr Shobha N Gudi** Bengaluru	**Dr Vidya Thobbi** Bijapur
Dr Vinita Singh Patna		

Contributors

Anshu Jindal MD DNB MNAMS
Clinical Director and Senior Consultant
Department of Reproductive Endocrinology
Jindal Hospital
Meerut, Uttar Pradesh, India

Asha R Rao MBBS MD (Obs & Gyne) FICOG
Infertility Specialist, Medical Director and
Chief Consultant
Department of Obstetrics and Gynecology
Rao Hospital and Centre for Assisted Reproduction and Endoscopy (CARE)
Coimbatore, Tamil Nadu, India

Fessy Louis T MBBBS DGO DNB MICOG FICOG
MNAMS DPS (Germany)
Professor and Head
Department of Reproductive Medicine
and Surgery
Amrita Fertility Centre
Amrita Institute of Medical Sciences (AIMS)
Kochi, Kerala, India
Past Vice President, FOGSI

JB Sharma MBBS MD
Professor
Department of Obstetrics and Gynecology
All India Institute of Medical Sciences
New Delhi, India
Chairperson, FOGSI Urogynecology
Committee

Madhuri Patil MD DGO FCPS DFP FICOG (Mum)
Clinical Director
Dr Patil's Fertility and Endoscopy Clinic
Bengaluru, Karnataka, India
Vice President, ISAR
President, Fertility
Preservation Society of India

Manasi Kamalakar Deoghare MBBS MD
Fellow Urogynecology
Department of Obstetrics and Gynecology
All India Institute of Medical Sciences
New Delhi, India

Poonam Goyal MD FICOG FICMCH CIMP
Director
Panchsheel Hospital
New Delhi, India
Head
Department of IVF and Infertility
Max Hospital, Vaishali, Delhi NCR
Chairperson
Safe Motherhood Committee, FOGSI
Governing Council Member, ICOG

Pragya Mishra Choudhary MBBS DFFP
MRCOG PhD FRCOG FICOG
Consultant Infertility Specialist
NuLife Test Tube Baby Centre, Patna
MGM Hospital and Research Centre
Patna, Bihar, India
Past Chairperson, FOGSI
Genetics and Fetal Medicine Committee

Pratik Tambe MD FICOG FICRM
ART Consultant and Gynec Endoscopic
Surgeon
Department of Obstetrics and Gynecology
Ashirwad IVF
Mumbai, Maharashtra, India
Governing Council Member, ICOG
(2020–2025)
Governing Council member, ICRM
(2024–2026)
Chairperson, AMOGS Endocrinology
Committee (2020–2024)
Chairperson, FOGSI Endocrinology
Committee (2017–2019)
Managing Council Member, MOGS,
ISAR, MSR

Seema Nishad
MCH Resident
Department of Reproductive Medicine
and Surgery
Amrita Fertility Centre
Amrita Institute of Medical Sciences (AIMS)
Kochi, Kerala, India

Sunil Jindal MS DNB MNAMS
Scientific Director and Senior Consultant
Department of Reproductive Medicine
Jindal Hospital
Meerut, Uttar Pradesh, India
Past Secretary, Delhi ISAR

Suyesha Khanijao MBBS DNB FNB
Director
Angel's Hope IVF
Sawan Neelu Angels Hospital
New Delhi, India

From the Desk of President, FOGSI

It gives me great pleasure to pen this message for the ICOG Campus issue on *Male Infertility* under the leadership of the Chairperson of ICOG, Dr Parul J Kotdawala; Vice Chairperson, Dr Sheela Mane; Secretary, Dr Sarita Bhalerao; Chairperson Elect, Dr Parag Biniwale; and Vice Chairperson Elect, Dr Ashok Kumar. The editors, Dr Pratik Tambe and Dr Asha R Rao have put together a comprehensive yet succinct issue on an important subject. I thank the authors Pragya Mishra Choudhary, Fessy Louis T, Poonam Goyal, JB Sharma, Sunil Jindal, Pratik Tambe, Madhuri Patil for their stellar efforts and hope that every member will use this as a valuable reference.

Warm regards,

Jaydeep Tank
President, FOGSI

FOGSI Secretary General's Message

Dear FOGSIans and ICOGians,
I bring greetings from the FOGSI!!

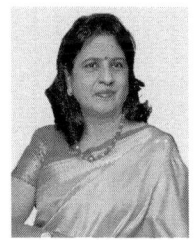

I am very pleased to know that the *ICOG Campus on Male Infertility* is being released soon.

The field of male infertility has witnessed significant advancements in recent years, with researchers and clinicians exploring new frontiers to better understand and address this complex condition. Male infertility is a condition which is quite widespread throughout the world and in our country but often does not receive the attention which it requires.

As our understanding of male infertility continues to evolve, the integration of newer concepts and current treatment methodologies into our clinical practice will be essential for improving the diagnosis, treatment and overall outcomes for men facing fertility challenges. This is essential if we are to keep up with modern advances and offer the best quality of care in our practices.

I congratulate Dr Jaydeep Tank, President, FOGSI and the ICOG Office Bearers Dr Parul J Kotdawala and Dr Sarita Bhalerao for envisioning such an important focused publication and the Editors Dr Pratik Tambe and Dr Asha R Rao for their hard work in ensuring that this was brought about in a very short space of time.

I have no doubt that the readers will find this publication very practical and useful as the contributors are some of the best clinicians in this field in India. I thank them for their timely submission and contributions. Ensuring good care practices and universal availability of health care is of paramount importance today and we as FOGSIans are dedicated toward the same!

Warm and personal regards,

M. A. Patel

Madhuri Patel
Secretary General, FOGSI
Editor-in-Chief, JOGI

From the Desk of Chairperson, ICOG

Dear Colleagues in ICOG and FOGSI,

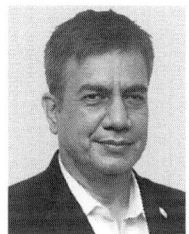

It gives me great pleasure to release the first ICOG Campus issue of the current year. The topic for the issue, *Male Infertility* is very important topic of current practice, as we observe a big rise in 'Male factor' in infertility management. All of us who have been dealing with fertility therapy for more than 3 decades have been wondering at the gradual rise in contribution of men as the cause of subfertility. Although many lifestyle factors are proposed to explain this curious phenomenon, the mystery remains unresolved.

The editors of this issue, Dr Pratik Tambe and Dr Asha R Rao have been quite successful in covering all aspects of this conundrum by collecting the latest updates from erudite authors. My sincere compliments to all the contributors to the Campus issue.

I join Dr Jaydeep Tank (President, FOGSI), Dr Madhuri Patel (Hon Secretary General, FOGSI) and my colleague in ICOG, Dr Sarita Bhalerao (Hon Secretary, ICOG) to put on records my appreciations and congratulations for the Editors (Dr Pratik Tambe and Dr Asha R Rao) for completing this challenging task at such a short notice. I also acknowledge the efforts and perseverance of the team of our publisher, M/s Jaypee Brothers Medical Publishers (P) Ltd, New Delhi, India.

I am very sure that this monograph will be very useful to all colleagues in their pursuits to help women and couples trying to get pregnant and the 'male factor' is the impediment.

Regards,

Parul J Kotdawala
Chairperson, ICOG

ICOG Vice Chairperson's Message

According to WHO, infertility affects one in 6 couples worldwide and about half of these cases can be attributed to male infertility.

There has been a rapid decline in male fertility in the past 2-3 decades. More men are being diagnosed with having low sperm counts and low motility abnormal morphology and also azoospermia.

Changes in lifestyle, rapid urbanization, environmental pollution, occupational hazards, smoking and stress can be the reason why many healthy young men in 20s and 30s are facing fertility issues.

In spite of advances in sperm function testing and surgical sperm retrieval techniques, male infertility still is neglected. The female partner is made to undergo a number of tests and procedures, but men do not get proper counseling and advice. It is time to understand that infertility consultation must be focused on both male and female partners. Men who face psychosexual problems often delay in seeking help. As we are spreading awareness about social egg freezing, men can also be encouraged to undergo testing soon after marriage to advise on lifestyles modification early on. We must understand that men also face societal pressure and mental health issues (as women) when they are unable to conceive a child.

Creating awareness and providing help and proper consultation is best way forward.

I am sure that this ICOG Campus on Male Infertility will enrich the knowledge of Obs/Gyne practitioners.

I congratulate Dr Pratik Tambe and Dr Asha R Rao for publicizing the ICOG Campus on Male Infertility.

Sheela Mane
Vice Chairperson, ICOG

ICOG Secretary's Message

Dear FOGSIans and ICOG Members,

Holi is just over, and we are just beginning our long hot summer season. Time to sit indoors and sip a cool drink and read. We bring you this year's first issue of ICOG Campus.

This issue is focused on a problem which is increasingly dominating our clinical practice—Male infertility. I congratulate Editors, Dr Pratik Tambe and Dr Asha R Rao for this excellent issue. They have covered all the important aspects from initial assessment to lifestyle factors and more sophisticated techniques of sperm retrieval. The authors are stalwarts in this field with many years of experience. I am certain you will find many practice points in this issue.

Our year started in January when the new ICOG team was installed at AICOG-2024 in Hyderabad. Under the dynamic leadership of Dr Parul J Kotdawala, ICOG webinars are being held every week. We did a very successful online certificate course on postpartum hemorrhage (PPH) curated by Dr Sheela Mane which was attended by more than 1000 delegates. Our first masterclass was held on polycystic ovarian disease (PCOD). The monthly journal club and research methodology meetings are popular with youngsters and senior practitioners. Postgraduate clinics on Sundays are a continuing feature from past years and continue to draw delegates.

ICOG training centers in Endoscopy, Reproductive Medicine and Fetal Medicine and others are doing tremendous work all over the country in training fresh graduates. The lecture series is exhaustive. I congratulate the center heads for this selfless work. As examiner, I was delighted to see these trainees so well informed and motivated. We encourage more students to take up these courses to enhance their skills.

We look forwards to seeing you all at the Annual ICOG Conference on October 19-21 in Ahmedabad. There will be a Membership and Fellowship convocation ceremony, 3 orations, many guest lectures, and workshops.

Happy reading and do visit *icogonline.org* for all recent updates!

Sarita Bhalerao
Secretary, ICOG

Preface

Dear Readers,

The Indian College of Obstetricians and Gynaecologists (ICOG) is the academic wing of FOGSI and has been in existence since 1984. It is the aim of the college to promote education and training and spread knowledge in the field of Obstetrics and Gynecology and related areas.

It is with great pride that we bring you the ICOG Campus on *Male Infertility: Recent Developments and Current Practice,* which focuses on an area which has seen tremendous research and great strides regarding management options.

In this publication, we focus on some of the most recent current evidence-based treatments in this field. We cover existing medications, newly introduced medical treatment alternatives and cutting-edge therapies including surgical management. The chapters have been authored by some of the foremost clinicians in the field and the readers will appreciate the focused content which will hopefully serve to improve their clinical practice.

We thank the ICOG Chairperson, Dr Parul J Kotdawala and Secretary Dr Sarita Bhalerao for giving us the opportunity to be part of such an innovative, important and immensely practical focused publication. We hope you enjoy reading the book and find it to be useful and impactful as regards day-to-day practice. We would welcome any comments or suggestions regarding the same and encourage you to reach out to us with feedback.

We would like to acknowledge the efforts of our publisher, M/s Jaypee Brothers Medical Publishers (P) Ltd, New Delhi, India, notably Ms Chetna Malhotra (Senior Director—Professional Publishing, Marketing, and Business Development) and Manpreet Kaur (Development Editor). We are also indebted to our academic partners who contributed generously, enabling us to print this volume and participated in the distribution of the same as well.

Wishing you, your families and staff good health and a Happy New Year!

Pratik Tambe
Asha R Rao
Editors

Contents

1. **Initial Assessment and Evaluation of Male Infertility** 1
   Asha R Rao

2. **Lifestyle Factors in Male Infertility** 8
   Pragya Mishra Choudhary

3. **Semen Investigations and Sperm Function Tests** 13
   Fessy Louis T, Seema Nishad

4. **Role of Imaging Modalities in Male Infertility** 20
   Poonam Goyal

5. **Surgical Management of Male Infertility** 28
   Manasi Kamalakar Deoghare, JB Sharma

6. **Sperm Retrieval Techniques** 33
   Sunil Jindal, Anshu Jindal

7. **Medical Management and Nutraceuticals** 43
   Pratik Tambe, Suyesha Khanijao

8. **Fertility Preservation in Men** 53
   Madhuri Patil

Index 65

Scan the QR code to access the Color Images.

Initial Assessment and Evaluation of Male Infertility

Asha R Rao

■ INTRODUCTION

Infertility has become a public health problem affecting approximately 1 in 10 couples globally. There are no reliable figures for global prevalence of infertility. It is estimated to be 8–12%, of which only the male partner accounts for 20%, females 38%, mixed 27%, and unknown 15%.[1] In India, it varies from 3.9 to 16.8% with wide variations not only in states but also in different tribes and castes of the same region.

The primary cause could be identified only in 40% of men with infertility. They are categorized as obstructive, nonobstructive, and coital factors. The reasons for most cases of (>75%) oligospermia remained unknown. There have been significant advances in male infertility over the past few decades, particularly in the development of novel diagnostic tools. Unfortunately, there remain a substantial number of patients who remain infertile despite these improvements.

■ GOALS OF MALE EVALUATIONS

There are several reasons for male infertility to occur, including both irreversible and reversible conditions. Other factors influencing each of the partners could be their age, medications, surgical history, exposure to environmental toxins, genetic problems, and systemic diseases.

The purpose of evaluating the male partner of a couple suffering from infertility is:
- To determine if the male factor is contributing to the infertility issue
- To offer treatment for those that are reversible
- To determine if assisted reproductive techniques (ARTs) would ultimately benefit the couple
- Offer counseling for irreversible and untreatable conditions

In rare cases, male infertility could be a herald to a more serious condition. This is an additional reason to do a comprehensive evaluation of the male partners of infertile couples; so that any significant, underlying medical conditions can be identified and treated.

INITIAL ASSESSMENT

- Infertility may be due to male factors, female factors, or both, hence a parallel evaluation of both partners is required.
- In couples with previous ART failures or recurrent pregnancy losses (RPLs), evaluation of the male factor should be considered (expert opinion).
- Initial evaluation of the male for fertility should include a complete and comprehensive sexual and medical history, including reproductive history and family history, trauma to pelvis/testicles, libido, sexual performance, occupation, intake of smoking/alcohol, recreational drugs, steroid abuse, pubertal development, previous radiotherapy/chemotherapy, testicular descent, surgical history involving the inguinal region and scrotum, sexually transmitted diseases, infections such as mumps/epididymitis, breast enlargement, and galactorrhea, and precocious puberty (≤9 years).
- Initial evaluation of the male should also include two or more semen analyses (strong recommendation; evidence level: Grade B). Perform semen analysis as per the WHO Laboratory Manual for the Examination and Processing of Human Semen (6th edition) reference criteria (strong recommendation) **(Table 1)**.[2]
- Men with one or more abnormal semen parameters should be evaluated by a male reproductive expert for a complete history and physical examination **(Flowchart 1)**.

TABLE 1: The lower reference limit for semen analysis.

Parameter 6th edition WHO lower reference limit	6th edition—5th centile data (95% CI)
Semen volume	>1.4 mL
Semen concentration × 10^6/mL	≥16 million
Total sperm no. × 10^6/ejaculation	≥39 million
TM (PR + NP)%	≥42%
PR%	≥30%
NP%	1%
IM%	20%
Vitality%	≥54%
Normal forms%	≥4.0%
Leukocytes	1–2 × 10^6/mL

(CI: confidence interval; IM: immotility; NP: nonprogressive motility; PR: progressive motility; TM: total motility)

Initial Assessment and Evaluation of Male Infertility

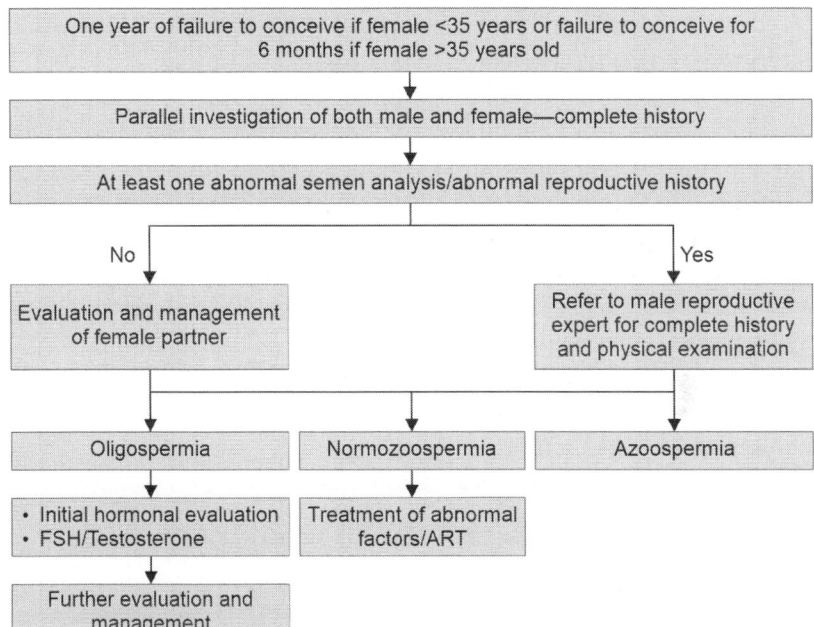

Flowchart 1: Initial evaluation of infertile couple.

(ART: assisted reproductive technique; FSH: follicle-stimulating hormone)

- In physical examination, look at the body form, possible signs of endocrinopathy, skin, hair distribution, gynecomastia, and secondary sexual characteristics.
- *Examination of penis*: Check for phimosis, hypospadias, and Peyronie plaques. The normal testicular volume in an adult male is 12–15 mL and length of the testis is 4 cm (<4 cm—small testis).
- The presence of vas deferens should be noted and documented [bilateral absent vas is reported in 1–2% of infertile men and it is associated with a mutation in *cystic fibrosis transmembrane conductance regulator (CFTR) gene*].[3]
- Presence or absence of hydrocele should be noted, and if present a testicular ultrasound should be used to examine the testis.
- Hypogonadism in childhood causes delayed puberty, in adults, erectile dysfunction, decreased libido, loss of secondary sexual characteristics, and infertility.
- Varicoceles are the most common correctable cause of male infertility, which is present in up to 15% of men and 40% in men with abnormal semen analysis. Clinically significant varicocele is generally believed to have an impact on infertility, but this remains controversial.[4] When present, they are typically seen on the left side due to anatomical reasons.

Isolated right-sided varicocele is suggestive of pathology in the retroperitoneal region, such as renal cell carcinoma (RCC) with an obstructing tumor thrombus in the vena cava.
- If the patient looks muscular with a low sperm count, do an endocrinological evaluation as he could have a low luteinizing hormone (LH) which is suggestive of testosterone abuse. Obese men will have low LH due to peripheral conversion of testosterone to estrogen which reduces LH, hence reduced sperm count.
- Infertile men with specific, identifiable causes of male infertility should be informed of relevant, associated health conditions (moderate recommendation; evidence level: Grade B).
- Clinicians should advise couples with advanced paternal age (>40 years) that there is an increased risk of adverse health outcomes for their offspring (expert opinion).
- Clinicians should discuss risk factors (i.e., lifestyle, medication usage, and environmental exposures) associated with male infertility (evidence level: Grade C).

■ DIAGNOSIS AND EVALUATION

- Semen analysis should be used to guide the management of the patient (expert opinion). At least two samples should be collected in a minimum interval of 1-4 weeks with <3 days of abstinence[5] (WHO 2- to 7-day abstinence recommendations appear to be arbitrary).
- *Hormonal evaluation* (**Table 2**):
  - Indicated in men with low sperm count and concentration (oligozoospermia or azoospermia) or with evidence of hormonal abnormality on physical evaluation, erectile dysfunction, impaired libido or atrophic testes (expert opinion).
  - Tests include follicle-stimulating hormone (FSH) and testosterone, LH, prolactin, thyroid-stimulating hormone (THS, optional), and estradiol (optional) levels [testosterone/estradiol (T/E) ratio <10 suggests a possible fertility benefit from an aromatase inhibitor to reduce the estrogen effect).
- Azoospermic men should be clinically evaluated to differentiate genital tract obstruction from impaired sperm production initially based on semen volume, physical examination, and FSH levels (expert opinion) (**Flowchart 2**).
- *Genetic screening and chromosomal testing:*
  - Karyotype and Y-chromosome microdeletion analysis should be recommended for men with primary infertility and azoospermia or severe oligozoospermia (<5 million sperm/mL)[6] (expert opinion).

TABLE 2: Male hormonal assay and its clinical interpretation.

FSH	LH	Testosterone	Interpretation	
Normal	Normal	Normal	Post-testicular absence/obstruction of vas/retrograde ejaculation	Semen analysis/physical findings
Low	Low	Low	Pretesticular (hypogonadotropic hypogonadism)	Karyotyping—central hypothalamo-pituitary forms
Normal/low	Normal/low	Low	Secondary hypogonadism	Check serum prolactin
High	Normal	Normal	Primary spermatogenic failure	Check testicular size/karyotyping/Y chromosome microdeletion
High	High	Low-normal	Primary testicular forms (spermatogenesis and Leydig cell damage)	Karyotyping/history chemotherapy

(FSH: follicle-stimulating hormone; LH: luteinizing hormone)

- Chromosomal abnormalities are more common in infertile men (15%) than in normal males (0.6%).
- Clinicians should recommend CFTR mutation carrier testing in men with absent vas deference or idiopathic obstructive azoospermia (expert opinion).[7]
- For men who harbor a CFTR mutation, genetic evaluation of the female partner should be recommended (expert opinion).
- Sperm deoxyribonucleic acid (DNA) fragmentation analysis is not recommended in the initial evaluation of the infertile couple (moderate recommendation; evidence level: Grade C). However, the test could be done in those with recurrent miscarriages.[8]
- Men with increased round cells on semen analysis (>1 million/mL) should be evaluated further to differentiate white blood cells (pyospermia) from germ cells (expert opinion).
- Patients with pyospermia should be evaluated for the presence of infection with sperm culture and sensitivity test (clinical principle).
- Antisperm antibody (ASA) testing should not be done in the initial evaluation of male infertility (expert opinion).
- For couples with RPL, men should be evaluated with karyotype (expert opinion) and sperm DNA fragmentation (moderate recommendation; evidence level: Grade C).

Flowchart 2: Evaluation of azoospermic male.

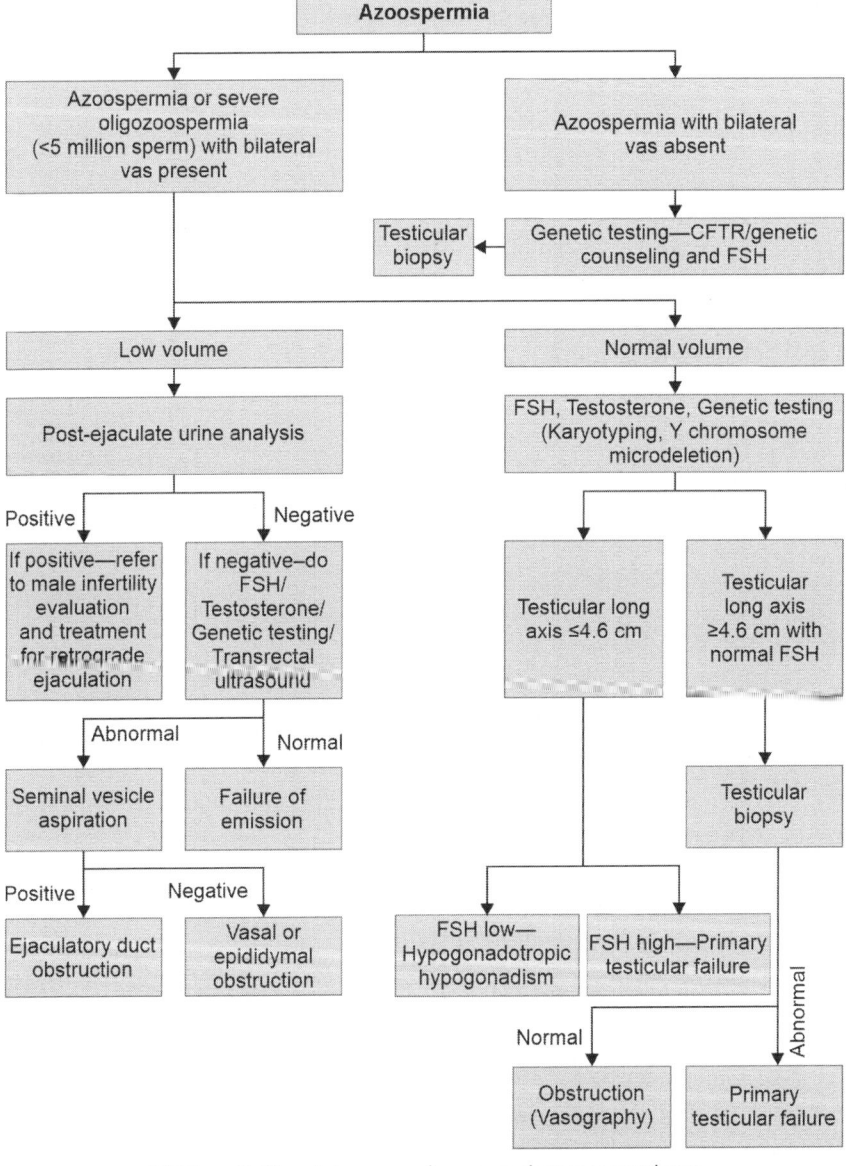

(CFTR: cystic fibrosis transmembrane conductance regulator; FSH: follicle-stimulating hormone)

- Diagnostic testicular biopsy should not routinely be performed to differentiate between obstructive azoospermia and nonobstructive azoospermia (NOA) (expert opinion).

IMAGING
- Scrotal ultrasound/transrectal ultrasonography (TRUS) should not be routinely performed in the initial evaluation of the infertile male (expert opinion).
- Clinicians should recommend TRUS in men with semen analysis suggestive of ejaculatory duct obstruction (i.e., acidic, azoospermic, semen volume <1.5 mL, with normal serum T, and palpable vas deferens) (expert opinion).
- Clinicians should recommend renal ultrasonography for patients with vasal agenesis to evaluate for renal abnormalities (expert opinion).

TESTICULAR BIOPSY
- Indicated to exclude spermatogenic failure.
- It is typically done in men suspected of ductal obstruction who present with azoospermia and normal hormonal screening tests and normal-sized testes.

CONCLUSION
A complete history, physical examination, and semen analysis are essential for initial evaluation of male infertility. More complex testing may be required in selected cases. Parallel evaluation of both male and female partners should be done to optimize treatment success.

REFERENCES
1. Winters BR, Walsh TJ. The epidemiology of male infertility. Urol Clin North Am. 2014;41(1):195-204.
2. Boitrelle F, Shah R, Saleh R, Henkel R, Kandil H, Chung E, et al. The Sixth Edition of the WHO Manual for Human Semen Analysis: A Critical Review and SWOT Analysis. Life (Basel). 2021;11(12):1368.
3. Patrizio P, Asch RH, Handelin B, Silber SJ. Aetiology of congenital absence of vas deferens: genetic study of three generations. Hum Reprod. 1993;8(2):215-20.
4. Kohn TP, Ohlander SJ, Jacob JS, Griffin TM, Lipshultz LI, Pastuszak AW. The effect of subclinical varicocele on pregnancy rates and semen parameters: a systematic review and meta-analysis. Curr Urol Rep. 2018;19(7):53.
5. Lotti F, Maggi M. Ultrasound of the male genital tract in relation to male reproductive health. Hum Reprod Update. 2015;21(1):56-83.
6. Ferlin A, Arredi B, Speltra E, Cazzadore C, Selice R, Garolla A, et al. Molecular and clinical characterization of Y chromosome microdeletions in infertile men: a 10-year experience in Italy. J Clin Endocrinol Metab. 2007;92(3):762-70.
7. Yu J, Chen Z, Ni Y, Li Z. CFTR mutations in men with congenital bilateral absence of the vas deferens (CBAVD): a systemic review and meta-analysis. Hum Reprod. 2012;27(1):25-35.
8. Zini A, Boman JM, Belzile E, Ciampi A. Sperm DNA damage is associated with an increased risk of pregnancy loss after IVF and ICSI: systematic review and meta-analysis. Hum Reprod. 2008;23(12):2663-8.

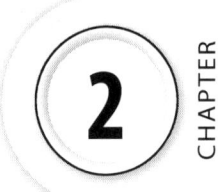

CHAPTER 2

Lifestyle Factors in Male Infertility

Pragya Mishra Choudhary

■ INTRODUCTION

There was a time when the cause for infertility or subfertility was ascribed only to the female partner, but now it is well proven that male factor is the primary or contributing cause in approximately 50% of cases. Undoubtedly, there has been a global decline in human sperm quality in the last few decades due to environmental, occupational, and lifestyle factors and in recent years, there has been growing interest in male lifestyle factors as the cause for infertility as these are modifiable to quite an extent.[1-3]

The common male lifestyle factors which are responsible for infertility are obesity, increased paternal age, undernutrition, cigarette smoking, alcohol, recreational drugs, coffee consumption, sedentary lifestyle, stress and depression, and use of mobile phones and laptops where there is a risk of electromagnetic radiation. Other modifiable lifestyle factors are testicular heat stress, intense cycling training, and lack of sleep.[2,3]

■ OBESITY

The incidence of obesity has tripled since the 1970s in reproductive age males and meta-analysis by Campbell et al. has shown that incidence of infertility is higher in couples with overweight partners compared to normal weight ones. The incidence of oligospermia and azoospermia is higher in men with greater body mass index (BMI). Systematic review of 30 studies comprising 115,158 males found that men who were obese had a higher percentage of sperm with deoxyribonucleic acid (DNA) fragmentation, abnormal morphology, and low mitochondrial membrane potential (MMP). A 14-week weight loss program has shown a decrease in cellular DNA damage and an increase in total motile sperm count.[4]

There are several theories behind obesity and male infertility. One is related to endocrinological abnormality of the hypothalamic–pituitary–gonadal axis. Increased aromatization of steroids to estrogen in the adipose tissue leads to a negative feedback mechanism, leading to hypogonadotropic hypogonadism with a significant reduction in total and free testosterone. Increase in estradiol and hyperinsulinemia in obese men leads to reduced sex hormone-binding globulin. There is a substantial decrease in inhibin B concentration which directly alters spermatogenesis and Sertoli cell function.

In obese men, there is a higher level of oxidative stress due to an imbalance between oxidants and antioxidants. Thermal effect due to increased scrotal adiposity can also harm the spermatocytes as proposed by some and lastly, the psychological impact can also lead to erectile dysfunction and reduced sexuality.[1]

■ CIGARETTE SMOKING AND SPERM QUALITY

The prevalence of smoking is very high in reproductive age men and nearly 37% men in this group smoke. The American Society for Reproductive Medicine (ASRM) once published that the quality of sperms in smokers is poorer than in nonsmokers. The hazardous chemicals from cigarette smoke are toxic to the sperm cells and can reduce the sperm count, motility, and morphology. The decline in semen quality has been found to be more marked in heavy (>20 cigarettes/day) and moderate (10-20 cigarettes/day) smokers compared to mild smokers (1-10 cigarettes/day).[2]

There are several theories to suggest what causes sperm quality to deteriorate in smokers. Cigarette smoke, which contains toxins, can damage the sperm chromatin structure, the sperm DNA, and decrease the sperm mitochondrial activity. It also leads to impaired acrosome reaction and capacitation and increased oxidative stress. In a study by Aboulmaouahib et al., sperm DNA fragmentation index (DFI) and sperm chromatin decondensation were significantly increased in smokers (25% and 23%), alcoholic (26% and 25%), and more for consumers of cigarette and alcohol (31% and 39%). Hypoxia resulting from cigarette smoke can also lead to impaired spermatogenesis and long-term cigarette smoking can lead to increased testosterone metabolism in the liver causing Sertoli and Leydig cell dysfunction. Subfertile males should be counseled to quit smoking or reduce the number of cigarettes smoked per day which can improve semen parameters.[3]

■ ALCOHOL INTAKE AND SEMEN QUALITY

Almost three decades ago, the first reports on the effects of alcohol intake on sperm quality and hormonal disorders were published. One of the first meta-analyses published in 2011 which included 29,914 participants found a significant relationship between alcohol intake, volume of semen, and both morphology and motility of semen. There was no effect of moderate drinking on sperm quality. The mechanisms which lead to the damaging impact of alcohol on male infertility could be due to an increased concentration of leukocytes in the seminal fluid and adverse effects on spermatogenesis. Alcohol-induced DNA damage is a result of increased reactive oxygen species. Hormonal changes are worse in daily drinkers compared to occasional drinkers. The ratio between free estradiol and free testosterone is modified by alcohol intake and spermatogenic arrest was found to be increasingly associated with high alcohol consumption. Time to pregnancy was longer in those couples where the male partner consumed >20 units per week. Male partners should be counseled to cut down on their alcohol intake.[4]

■ RECREATIONAL DRUGS

Illicit drug use such as marijuana, cocaine, anabolic-androgenic steroids (AAS), opiates, and methamphetamines lead to a negative impact on male infertility. These drugs affect the hypothalamic–pituitary–gonadal axis. Marijuana smoking more than once weekly has been known to reduce the sperm count and concentration and this effect can be further exacerbated with multirecreational drug use. Both acute and chronic exposure to cocaine can damage the testicular ultrastructure and affect spermatogenesis. Males who have indulged in long-term cocaine use have a lower sperm count, concentration, and higher fraction of sperms with abnormal morphology. These men should be strongly encouraged to join drug rehabilitation centers.

Use of AAS is on the rise not only by professional athletes but also by young men and teenagers to enhance their personal appearance. Use of AAS can lead to anabolic steroid-induced hypogonadism (testosterone <50 ng/mL) with reversible suppression of spermatogenesis, testicular atrophy, and infertility. Use of AAS should be strongly discouraged.[2]

■ EFFECTS OF MOBILE PHONES AND PORTABLE COMPUTERS ON SEMEN QUALITY

There has been a recent concern about the use of mobile phones and portable computers as a source of low-level radiofrequency electromagnetic field (RF-EMF). A meta-analysis by Adams et al. reported that there is a relationship between use of mobile phones and reduction in sperm motility and vitality but not sperm concentration. Another meta-analysis by Hieu et al. reported that mobile phone usage did not have an effect on semen parameters. Some authors have independently reported that men who carry mobile phones in their pant pockets have a higher incidence of sperm DFI compared to those who carry mobile phones in their shirt pockets.[3]

■ STRESS

Stress can be a cause of both male and female infertility. Stress can activate the hypothalamic–pituitary–adrenal (HPA) axis which inhibits the hypothalamic–pituitary–gonadal axis and suppresses testosterone secretion. Reduction of testosterone levels acts upon the Leydig cells and the testis blood-brain barrier and spermatogenesis is suppressed. Studies have investigated the association between psychological stress in the form of occupational stress, life stress, family functioning, examination stress, and semen quality. Most of them have shown psychological stress to be associated with reduced paternity and abnormal semen parameters. Men should be counseled regarding stress factor in infertility and self-measures to alleviate stress out of their lives.[1,4]

ADVANCED PATERNAL AGE

As age increases, there are changes in testicular morphology and structure, such as a decrease in the number of germ cells and Sertoli-Leydig cells, narrowing of seminiferous tubules as a result of which testicular function and metabolism deteriorates leading to a decline in total sperm count, progressive motility, and the percentage of normal forms. With age, there is also an increase of reactive oxygen species and sperm DNA fragmentation. Overall sperm quality declines with age and advanced paternal age (APA) is also related to spontaneous pregnancy loss and negative pregnancy outcomes. Hence, couples should be equally emphasized regarding the contribution of APA and advanced maternal age (AMA) toward reduced fertility and poor reproductive outcome.[2]

DIET

A very important aspect of male lifestyle factor is having a balanced diet rich in vitamins and antioxidants. In this regard, a Mediterranean diet which contains more fruits, green vegetables, whole grains, and white meat and is rich in omega-3 fatty acids is considered superior to a western diet with red meat, processed cheese, refined grains, and high-energy drinks. Men should be encouraged to go for a more prudent diet avoiding processed meat, full-fat dairy products, alcohol, coffee, and sugar-sweetened beverages which are associated with poor semen parameters and reduced fecundity rates.[3]

OTHER LIFESTYLE FACTORS

Other lifestyle factors such as sleep disturbances, use of electronic gadgets, prolonged hours of sitting, and exposure to radiant heat can all have a profound effect on sperm count as has been shown by some studies. In addition, tight undergarments, sauna baths, and long-distance cycling may all cause spermatozoal abnormalities by creating scrotal hyperthermia and trauma.[2]

CONCLUSION

There has been a progressive decline in semen quality of men worldwide, which has led to lower semen parameters in the World Health Organization (WHO) 5th and 6th editions. It is high time that subfertile men be educated and counseled about modifiable lifestyle factors which play an important role in the causation and further deterioration of male subfertility.[1-4]

REFERENCES

1. Chakravarty BN (Ed). Evaluation of male infertility. Clinics in Reproductive Medicine and Assisted Reproductive Technology, 1st edition. New Delhi: CBS Publishers & Distributors Pvt Ltd; 2015. pp. 1-15.
2. Balawender K, Orkisz S. The impact of selected modifiable lifestyle factors on male fertility in the modern world. Cent European J Urol. 2020;73(4):563-8.
3. Durairajanayagam D. Lifestyle causes of male infertility. Arab J Urol. 2018;16(1):10-20.
4. Agarwal A, Baskaran S, Parekh N, Cho CL, Henkel R, Vij S, et al. Male Infertility. Lancet. 2021;397(10271):319-33.

CHAPTER 3
Semen Investigations and Sperm Function Tests

Fessy Louis T, Seema Nishad

INTRODUCTION

In infertile couples, male factor is solely responsible in approximately 20% of cases and involved as contributory factor in another 30–40% of cases. Thus, male factor can be considered as cause in nearly half of all infertility cases.[1] Most important and basic investigation for evaluating the functioning of male reproductive organs is semen analysis. The World Health Organization (WHO) provides manual for semen analysis and other laboratory tests to evaluate male partner.

SEMEN ANALYSIS

It is the most basic test. Semen specimen is collected by masturbation into a clean, dry, sterile, and wide mouth container or if masturbation is not possible then during coitus using special condoms (containing no spermicidal lubricants). The WHO published reference ranges for semen testing in 2021.[2] These include "lower reference limits" representing the 5th percentiles for semen characteristics. Point to remember is that the lower reference limits do not serve as a cut-off point between "fertile" and "infertile". The European Association of Urology (EAU) guidelines recommend to repeat semen analysis after 4–6 weeks in case of abnormal results.

Parameters examined in the semen analysis and their lower reference limits are given in **Table 1**.

Volume

About 90% of the volume of semen is composed of secretions from the accessory organs, mainly the prostate and seminal vesicles with minor contributions from the bulbourethral (Cowper's) glands and epididymides. Decreased volume can be due to obstructive pathology. Anejaculation (absence of ejaculate) can be due to retrograde ejaculation. Semen analysis 6th edition states that information of a strong odor of urine or putrefaction can be of clinical importance.[3]

pH of Semen

Prostatic secretion is acidic and seminal vesicular secretion is alkaline. A pH value under 7.2 may be indicative of a lack of alkaline seminal vesicular fluid. It can also be due to urine contamination.

TABLE 1: Parameters examined in the semen analysis and their lower reference limits.[2]

Parameters	Lower reference limits	
	WHO 2010	WHO 2021
Abstinence	2–7 days	2–7 days
Volume	1.5 mL	1.4 mL
Sperm concentration (×10^6/mL)	15	16
Total sperm count (×10^6/ejaculation)	39	39
Total motility (%)	40	42
Progressive motility (%)	32	30
Nonprogressive motility (%)	1	1
Immotile (%)	22	20
Vitality (%)	58	54
Normal forms (%)	4	4
Leukocytes (million/mL)	>1	>1

(WHO: World Health Organization)

Seminal Fructose

The normal value for seminal fructose level is >13 μmol/mL. Fructose is absent in semen in cases with absence of vas deferens or ejaculatory duct obstruction (EDO).

Total Sperm Count

Total number of spermatozoa ejaculated (sperm concentration multiplied by semen volume) is a better reflection of the capacity for sperm production.

Sperm Concentration

Sperm concentration is the number of sperm/mL in a semen sample. Oligospermia is a decrease in the sperm concentration in semen below 15 million sperm per milliliter (WHO, 2010). It is severe oligospermia if <5 million/mL.

Total Motile Sperm Count

Total motile sperm count (TMSC) is obtained by multiplying the volume of the ejaculate in milliliters by the sperm concentration and the proportion of A (fast forward progressive) and B (slow progressive) motile sperms, divided by 100%.

Sperm Vitality

It is not necessary when at least 40% of spermatozoa are motile. Vitality test is important to discriminate between immotile dead sperm and immotile live sperm. Immotile cells may be indicative of structural defects in the flagellum. High percentage of immotile and dead cells may indicate epididymal pathology or an immunological reaction due to an infection.

Sperm Morphology

Assessment of sperm morphology is done by assessment of head, neck, and midpiece, and tail of sperms. Decreased count of sperms with normal morphology (teratospermia) is associated with subfertility. Treatment would be assisted reproductive technique (ART), possibly in vitro fertilization (IVF) with intracytoplasmic sperm injection (ICSI). Selection of sperms can be done by various methods to perform ICSI.

Sperm Motility

Low motility (asthenozoospermia) can be managed by giving antioxidants followed by intrauterine insemination (IUI) and in severe cases, ART with ICSI can be done.

Leukocytes

Levels above 1 million/mL in the semen are considered excessive (pyospermia or leukospermia) and possibly indicative of infection. It has been suggested that excessive numbers of leukocytes in the semen could contribute to infertility by the release of free radicals from the neutrophils resulting in oxidative damage to the sperm.

Postejaculatory Urine Analysis

It is recommended in cases of anejaculation (no ejaculate after orgasm), as presence of sperms in urine after masturbation may be required to confirm retrograde ejaculation. Collected sperms can be used for IVF with ICSI.

■ PHYSICAL EXAMINATION

If patient has abnormal semen analysis parameters or any sexual dysfunction, physical examination of male partner is needed. During the physical examination, it is important to check for possible signs of endocrinopathy, gynecomastia, skin, hair distribution, and particularly secondary sexual characteristics.[4] Obesity tends to increase the peripheral conversion of testosterone to estrogen.

Testicular size reflects the level of spermatogenic capacity. Testicular size should be measured. In a normal adult male, the testicular volume should be at least 15 mL, and the length of the testis should be at least 4 cm. Mild painful sensation to touch to testis is normal, but exquisite tenderness can be due to torsion or infection.

The bilateral absence of the vas is reported in 1–2% of infertile men and is related to mutations of the *cystic fibrosis transmembrane conductance regulator (CFTR)* gene, even in the absence of any clinical signs of cystic fibrosis.[5]

The presence of a hydrocele and varicocele should be noted. Varicoceles are the most common correctable cause of male infertility. Large size of testis can be a suspicious finding for presence of hydrocele. Varicocele can be palpated, in standing position, as bag of worms at neck of scrotum. Findings can be confirmed by scrotal ultrasound.

Examination of the penis would include a check for hypospadias, phimosis, and Peyronie plaques.

■ HORMONAL EVALUATION

Hormonal evaluation is indicated if there is a low sperm concentration (<10 million/mL) or azoospermia, clinical findings suggestive of endocrine disorder or impaired sexual function. The endocrine laboratory test panel would include serum follicle-stimulating hormone (FSH), testosterone, luteinizing hormone (LH), prolactin, thyroid-stimulating hormone (TSH), and estradiol levels[6] **(Table 2)**.

- Hypergonadotropic hypogonadism affects both sperm production and testosterone levels. Karyotyping should be performed.
- Primary spermatogenic failure, especially if associated with azoospermia or severe oligozoospermia. Check testicular size and consider karyotyping as well as Y chromosome microdeletion testing.
- Cushing's disease (buffalo hump, moon face, etc.) diagnosed by a 24-hour urine test for free cortisol, a dexamethasone suppression test, or by checking the midnight salivary cortisol concentration.
- Thyroid dysfunction can be identified by abnormal serum thyroid function tests.
- *Hyperprolactinemia:* High prolactin level may be associated with thyroid dysfunction or can cause male sexual dysfunction.

TABLE 2: Hormonal evaluation.

	Secondary hypogonadism	Obstructive azoospermia	Hypergonadotropic hypogonadism	Primary spermatogenic failure	Partial androgen resistance
FSH	Normal/low	Normal	High	High	Normal
LH	Normal/low	Normal	High	Normal	High
Testosterone	Low	Normal	Low	Normal	High

(FSH: follicle-stimulating hormone; LH: luteinizing hormone)

IMAGING INVESTIGATIONS

Scrotal ultrasound and transrectal ultrasonography (TRUS) should not be routinely performed in the initial evaluation of the infertile male.[7]

If a hydrocele is suspected on clinical examination, a scrotal ultrasound can be used to confirm. Clinicians should recommend TRUS in men with suggestive of EDO (i.e., acidic, aspermia, or azoospermic, semen volume <1.5 mL, with normal serum testosterone, and palpable vas deferens).[4]

SPERM FUNCTION TESTS

Antisperm Antibodies

Antisperm antibodies (ASAs) should be suspected with sperm agglutination or isolated asthenozoospermia with normal sperm concentrations. These antibodies can be formed due to testicular surgery or vasectomy, prostatitis or anytime sperm comes into contact with blood. ASA testing should not be done in the initial evaluation. Antibodies can be tested by postcoital test, mixed antiglobulin reaction (MAR) test, immunobead test, etc.[4]

Sperm Vitality Tests

Vitality is estimated by assessing the membrane integrity of the cells. Vitality can be tested by eosin staining, eosin-nigrosin staining, and hypo-osmotic swelling test (HOS test). If >25–30% of all spermatozoa are alive and immotile, a genetic ciliary problem may be the cause.[4]

Deoxyribonucleic Acid Integrity Test

Deoxyribonucleic acid (DNA) integrity test assesses the degree of sperm DNA fragmentation (SDF). SDF tests can be considered in patients with varicocele, unexplained infertility, IUI failure or recurrent implantation failure, etc. A variety of techniques have been developed to assess the integrity of sperm DNA material. If DNA fragmentation index (DFI) assessed by sperm chromatin structure assay (SCSA) exceeds the threshold value of 30%, ICSI should be indicated in these couples.[8]

Capacitation, Acrosomal Reaction, and Sperm Penetration Assays[4]

Used for cases where a sperm defect is suspected, as in cases where IUI has repeatedly failed. IVF with ICSI is the preferred treatment for men whose sperm show poor results on any of these tests.

Reactive Oxygen Species

Spermatozoa are particularly susceptible to reactive oxygen species (ROS)-induced damage compared to other cells. ROS production is positively correlated with the proportion of sperm with morphologically deformed sperms and leukocytes. ROS include superoxide anions, hydrogen peroxide, hydroxyl radicals, nitric oxide, etc. Nitroblue tetrazolium test and chemiluminescence test can also be done by using probes.[9]

GENETIC EVALUATION

Genetic tests are typically recommended for patients with severe oligozoospermia (<5 million sperm/mL) or azoospermia as chromosomal defects are more common in infertile men (up to 15%) than in normal males (about 0.6%). Genetic tests consist of karyotype, CFTR, and Y chromosome testing for microdeletions.[10] The common genetic factors associated with infertility in males are impaired testicular function due to chromosomal abnormalities (Klinefelter syndrome), isolated spermatogenic impairment due to Y chromosome microdeletions, and congenital absence of the vas deferens due to *CFTR* gene mutation.[5] While ICSI can help these men with defective genes to father children, but they should be counseled for associated increased risk of transmission of various genetic defects to the progeny.

Congenital bilateral absence of the vas deferens (CBAVD) on physical examination is associated with *CFTR* gene mutations, and both partners should be genetically checked.[5] If a positive result is found, genetic counseling should be done prior to ARTs ICSI.

CONCLUSION

In all subfertile couples, initial evaluation must include male partner's physical examination and semen analysis. In cases of detected abnormalities during initial evaluation, subsequent investigations are warranted to ascertain underlying factors and facilitate appropriate management.

REFERENCES

1. Infertility Workup for the Women's Health Specialist: ACOG Committee Opinion, number 781. Obstet Gynecol. 2019;133:e377.
2. World Health Organization Laboratory Manual for the Examination and Processing of Human Semen, Sixth Edition, 2021.
3. Chung E, Atmoko W, Saleh R, Shah R, Agarwal A. Sixth Edition of the World Health Organization Laboratory Manual of Semen Analysis: Updates and Essential Take Away for Busy Clinicians. Arab J Urol. 2023;22(2):71-4.
4. Practice Committee of the American Society for Reproductive Medicine. Diagnostic evaluation of the infertile male: a committee opinion. Fertil Steril. 2015;103(3):e18-25.
5. Bieth E, Hamdi SM, Mieusset R. Genetics of the congenital absence of the vas deferens. Hum Genet. 2021;140:59-76.

6. Ross A, Bhasin S. Hypogonadism: its prevalence and diagnosis. Urol Clin North Am. 2016;43(2):163-76.
7. Kose SI. Imaging in Male Infertility. Current Problems in Diagnostic Radiology. 2023;52(5);439-47.
8. Leslie SW, Soon-Sutton TL, Khan MAB. StatPearls [Internet]. Male Infertility. StatPearls Publishing; Treasure Island (FL): Mar 3, 2023.
9. Takalani NB, Monageng EM, Mohlala K, Monsees TK, Henkel R, Opuwari CS. Role of oxidative stress in male infertility. Reproduction and Fertility. 2023;4(3):e230024.
10. Vander Borght M, Wyns C. Fertility and infertility: definition and epidemiology. Clin Biochem. 2018;62:2-10.

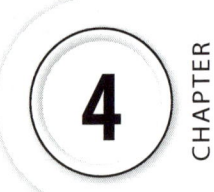

Role of Imaging Modalities in Male Infertility

CHAPTER 4

Poonam Goyal

■ INTRODUCTION

Infertility is delineated herein as the incapacity to attain pregnancy following recurrent participation in unprotected sexual intercourse for a duration of 1 year. Amidst couples experiencing infertility, the etiology often times implicates the male counterpart in roughly half of the cases. In 20% of infertile couples, male partner is the culprit. Male infertility typically ensues from conditions impacting spermiogenesis, sperm functionality, or both, as well as obstructions impeding sperm transport. In fact, male infertility is a multifaceted condition affecting millions worldwide and is on the increase due to stress, dietary habits, environmental factors, and substance abuse.

Traditional semen analysis remains the most fundamental diagnostic tool, but the integration of advanced imaging modalities has revolutionized our understanding and management of male infertility by casting light upon the intricate anatomical, physiological, and pathological nuances that underlie the male reproductive dysfunction.

In this chapter, we shall delve into the pivotal role of imaging methods offering insight to assisted reproductive technique (ART) specialists and other clinicians navigating this complex landscape of male infertility.

■ EVALUATION OF MALE INFERTILITY WITH IMAGING MODALITIES

After history, physical examination, and semen analysis if anything is found to be abnormal next step in work-up is to resort to imaging modalities.
- Ultrasonography (USG)
- Magnetic resonance imaging (MRI)
- Computed tomography (CT) scan
- Vasography
- Venography

■ ROLE OF IMAGING

- *Anatomical evaluation:* Imaging techniques such as USG and MRI play vital role in assessing the structural integrity. MRI complements USG by providing superior soft tissue contrast.

- *Vascular assessment:* Doppler ultrasound (US) is a very valuable tool in judging and quantifying the vascular perfusion with in male reproductive tract. Blood flow dynamics aids in diagnosis of varicocele. Perception of ejaculatory function can also be done.
- *Functional insights:* Beyond anatomical detailing, imaging offers insight into physiological aspects relevant to male infertility.

Imaging can be helpful as a guide for impregnating the female partner such as embryo transfer and intrauterine insemination (IUI). It ensures the right place to deposit sperms and embryos.

ULTRASOUND IN MALE INFERTILITY

Ultrasound is almost always the first step in imaging workup. Assessment is mainly meant for evaluating the testicular morphology, peritesticular structures prostatic anomalies, and judging patency of efferent ducts and varicocele with assessment of functional capacity. With scrotal USG and transrectal ultrasound (TRUS) scan almost the entire genital tract can be assessed, it helps in differentiation of obstructive from nonobstructive azoospermia (NOA). Obstruction can be there at in any point along the ductal system.[1]

Scrotal Ultrasonography

It is excellent favored modality for initial assessment owing to its noninvasiveness, safety, and cost-effectiveness. It is done in supine position. This diagnostic approach proves instrumental in scrutinizing potential testicular anomalies, gauging testicular volume, and detecting peritesticular irregularities such as varicocele, epididymal, and prostatic abnormalities. Employing a high frequency (7–12 MHz) linear array transducer, scrotal US entails transverse, orthogonal, and longitudinal assessment of the testes, complemented by color flow Doppler US to delineate testicular and spermatic cord vascularity. Essential to this evaluation are testicular volume measurements which are calculated via (length × width × anteroposterior diameter) normal volume ranges between 12–15 mL. Normal testis will have uniform regular echogenicity showing smoothness **(Fig. 1A)**. Whereas abnormal testis will be small and will have coarse echogenicity **(Fig. 1B)** and microcalcifications.[2]

In obstructive azoospermia (OA), there is retention of secretions leading to macroscopic changes proximal to obstruction. These secondary signs are ectasia of rete testis and dilated epididymal ductules. Enlarged testicular volume is there due to intratesticular cysts.[3]

In individuals diagnosed with congenital bilateral absence of the vas deferens (CBAVD), scrotal US reveals dilated efferent ducts with the epididymis terminating abruptly at the junction of the body and tail, beyond

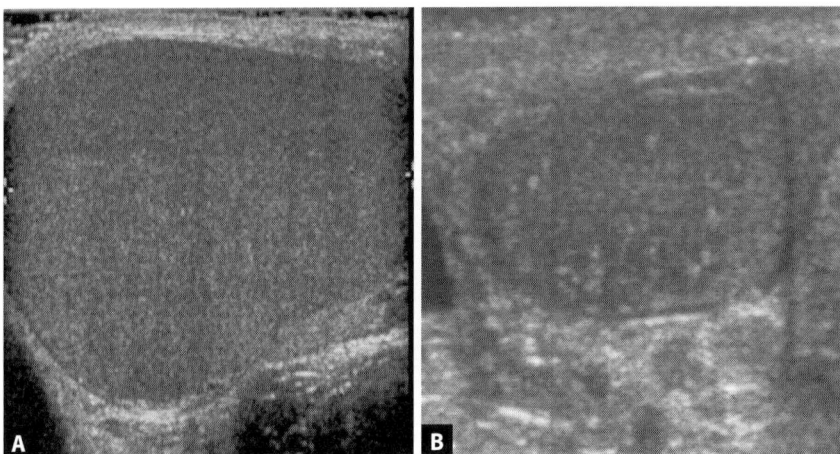

Figs. 1A and B: (A) Normal testis; (B) Small testis with coarse echogenicity.

which the vas deferens is absent. Epididymal isolated cysts maybe seen in normal men but if multiple it suggests obstruction.

Primary testicular tumors, notably germ cell tumors, are linked to reduced semen quality and fertility. Scrotal US aids in their assessment, revealing heterogeneous and low-reflectivity masses with increased vascularity.[3] Early detection and preservation of semen pretherapy are crucial considerations in testicular cancer management.

Testicular atrophy, resulting from various factors including inflammation and aging, manifests as global testicular volume reduction on US.

Even the failure of testicular descent into the scrotal sac is the most common congenital abnormality, impacting spermatogenesis and increasing the risk of malignancy.

Transabdominal Ultrasound

It should be done routinely for assessing the genital tract as well as for renal assessment.

It is done in left lateral decubitus position using a high frequency endorectal probe. It serves as a viable option for prostate evaluation, terminal vas deference, seminal vesicles (SVs), and ejaculatory duct (ED) thus potentially uncovering central sources resulting in spermatic obstruction.[4] A SV diameter surpassing 1.5 cm and an ED diameter exceeding 2.3 mm are suggestive of ED obstruction more so if it is in association with small cysts (**Fig. 2**) or microcalcifications.[5,6] TRUS has been recognized as an important diagnostic tool in the assessment of azoospermia, chiefly when associated with low ejaculate volume.[7,8] TRUS is currently found to be more sensitive in detecting OA than scrotal US.[9]

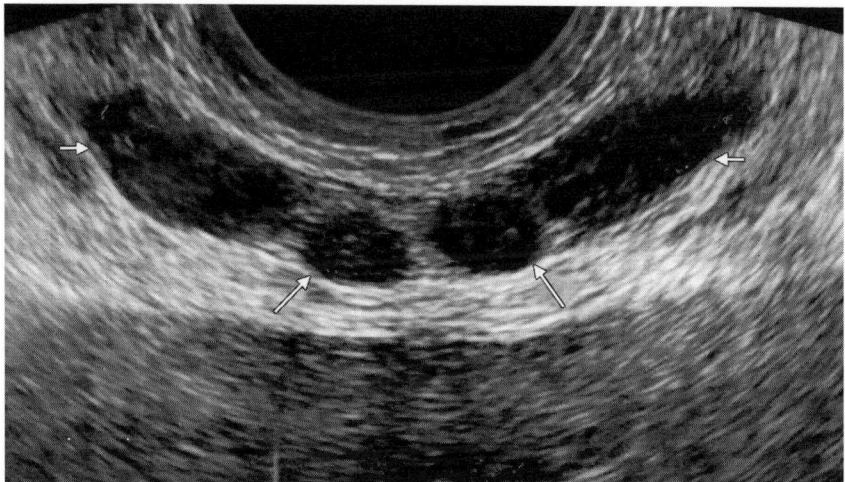

Fig. 2: Transrectal ultrasound (TRUS) image of seminal vesicles (small arrows) and medially vasa deferentia.

It was found that dilation of the ED was the most common cause of OA, followed by SV abnormalities and congenital abnormalities. TRUS is consistent and suitable method for diagnosing agenesis or hypoplasia of the SV in OA cases.[10]

Penile Ultrasound

Penile US serves as a pivotal tool in assessing the physical etiologies of erectile dysfunction. These encompass structural penile irregularities, disturbances in arterial blood flow, and malfunctions in the venous occlusive mechanism.[11] The evaluation commences with grayscale US to rule out structural abnormalities, such as fibrotic plaque diseases, focal cavernosal fibrosis or calcification, and tunica albuginea disruption.[12]

Subsequently, intracavernosal injection of prostaglandin E1 (PGE1) is administered. Placing the transducer on the ventral surface of the penile base, Doppler angle correction facilitates accurate velocity measurements of the cavernosal artery **(Fig. 3)**. Peak systolic velocity and end-diastolic velocity (EDV) are monitored at 5-minute intervals post-PGE1 injection, extending up to 30 minutes.

■ DOPPLER STUDY[3]

The pre-eminent culprit behind amendable male infertility is none other than the varicocele. These vascular anomalies, most elegantly unveiled through the grayscale and Doppler sonography, present as internal spermatic veins

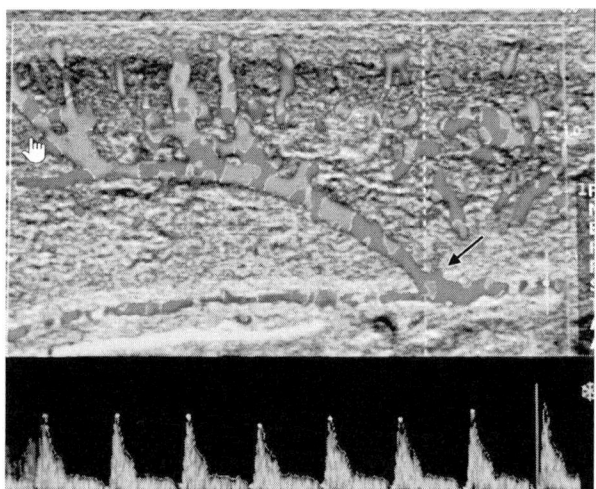

Fig. 3: Cavernosal artery on Doppler sonography. *(For color version, see Plate 1).*

luxuriously dilated beyond the threshold of 3 mm.[3] Employing the Valsalva maneuver allows examination of vein dynamics under the crescendo of abdominal pressure.[3] Varicoceles are the culprit in 40% of men afflicted with primary infertility and an astonishing 45–80% of secondary infertility.[3] Clandestine varicosity can cause infertility. On gray scale also, it is seen as serpiginous structure on posterior aspect of testis with two or three veins of pampiniform plexus measuring >2–3 mm in diameter.

■ MAGNETIC RESONANCE IMAGING[1]

The keen eye captures the details of testicular architecture with unparalleled finesse. MRI can give much better soft tissue contrast and such revelation is invaluable, particularly in cases of suspected neoplasms or congenital anomalies where clarity is of paramount importance.

- In imaging pituitary for micro- and macroadenomas.
- In localization of undescended testis in abdomen.

Anomalies such as prostatic urethra cysts and cystic dilatation of the prostatic utricle are challenging to distinguish on TRUS. MRI aids in characterization. A pelvic body coil is used or endorectal coils for better imaging. The use of endorectal coil requires bowel preparation **(Figs. 4A to D)**. In conclusion, while US remains the stalwart guardian of male infertility evaluation, MRI assumes its rightful place as a distinguished adjunct, wielding its unique capabilities to illuminate the hidden recesses anatomy and pathology with a moderate yet undeniable flair for the fanciful.[1]

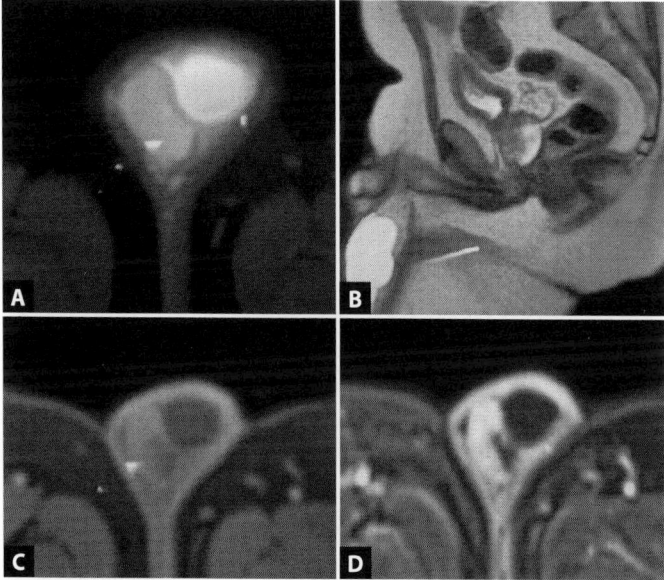

Figs. 4A to D: Magnetic resonance imaging (MRI) image of testis and scrotum.

■ COMPUTED TOMOGRAPHY SCAN[3]

Computed tomography enables limited soft tissue resolution and is used less often to evaluate infertility. CT is most useful for assessing calcifications and stones along the reproductive tract that may lead to obstruction.

■ VASOGRAPHY[3]

It is for vasal study. Once considered the reference standard for evaluating the male reproductive system, vasography, also known as seminal vesiculography, involves cannulation of the vas deferens under anesthesia. Owing to the prevalent acceptance of MRI, this invasive examination is no longer used to assess the male reproductive system. At present, vasography may be done to diagnose aplasia or occlusion of the EDs in males with azoospermia who are found to have normal spermatogenesis at testicular biopsy. This technique involves risk for infection and strictures of the vas deferens at the injection site.

■ VENOGRAPHY[1]

It is taken as gold standard for diagnosing varicocele by demonstrating reflux of contrast into testicular vein.[1] But it is invasive, and approach is from femoral vein usually. Mostly the varicocele is in the left testicular vein which drains in left renal vein and right drains directly in inferior vena cava (IVC).

Once the hydrophilic catheter is in place check venogram is done. We have to take care of collateral, if any.

■ NEW IN HORIZON

Currently work is being done on the study of various neurological tracts which are responsible for erectile function by fMRI, i.e., functional MRI. It measures the small changes in blood flow that occur with brain activity.

■ CONCLUSION

The thorough investigation of male infertility is paramount, aiming to unveil potentially remediable factors and steer therapeutic interventions. Central to this diagnostic journey is the crucial differentiation between NOA and OA. The integration of advanced imaging modalities has become indispensable, with scrotal US serving as an initial discriminator between OA and NOA, while subsequent techniques such as TRUS and MRI provide detailed delineation of obstruction levels, often elucidating underlying etiologies in cases of OA. Notably, scrotal US findings can instigate targeted interventions, be it the correction of varicocele, addressing testicular maldescent, or pursuing further evaluation in suspected cases of testicular tumors. Imaging plays a key role in the evaluation of the hypospermic or azoospermic man. It can diagnose reversible abnormalities that can be corrected, which can thereby lead to a fruitful conception.

Upon identifying findings suggestive of OA via scrotal US, a natural progression entails TRUS examination to discern proximal from distal obstruction. For patients with proximal obstruction, the option of vasoepididymostomy may be considered. Conversely, in cases of distal obstruction, additional imaging studies, such as TRUS or MRI, play a pivotal role in identifying potential urogenital cysts, amenable to US-guided aspiration albeit with often transient efficacy. Furthermore, US-guided sperm retrieval emerges as a viable approach. Should cystic pathology be absent, transurethral resection of the EDs stands as a plausible intervention, predicated upon the presumption of distal ductal anomalies contributing to obstructive pathology.

■ REFERENCES

1. Ammar T, Sidhu PS, Wilkins CJ. Male infertility: the role of imaging in diagnosis and management. Br J Radiol. 2012;85 Spec No 1(Spec Iss 1):S59-68.
2. Sihag P, Tandon A, Pal R, Jain BK, Bhatt S, Kaur S, et al. Sonography in male infertility: a look beyond the obvious. J Ultrasound. 2018;21(3):265-76.
3. Mittal PK, Little B, Harri PA, Miller FH, Alexander LF, Kalb B, et al. Role of imaging in the evaluation of male infertility. Radiographics. 2017;37(3):837-54.

4. Cocuzza M, Cardoso JP, Parekattil SJ. Imaging modalities in the management of male infertility. In: Parekattil S, Esteves S, Agarwal A (Eds). Male Infertility, 2nd edition. Germany: Springer; 2020.
5. Edey AJ, Sidhu PS. Male infertility: role of imaging in the diagnosis and management. Imaging. 2008;20:139-46.
6. Schurich M, Aigner F, Frauscher F, Pallwein L. The role of ultrasound in assessment of male fertility. Eur J Obstet Gynecol Reprod Biol. 2009;144(Suppl 1): S192-8.
7. Donkol RH. Imaging in male-factor obstructive infertility. World J Radiol. 2010; 2:172-9.
8. Worischeck JH, Parra RO. Transrectal ultrasound in the evaluation of men with low volume azoospermia. J Urol. 1993;149:1341-4.
9. Raviv G, Mor Y, Levron J, Shefi S, Zilberman D, Ramon J, et al. Role of transrectal ultrasonography in the evaluation of azoospermic men with low-volume ejaculate. J Ultrasound Med. 2006;25:825-9.
10. Abdulwahed SR, Mohamed EE, Taha EA, Saleh MA, Abdelsalam YM, ElGanainy EO. Sensitivity and specificity of ultrasonography in predicting etiology of azoospermia. Urology. 2013;81:967-71.
11. Raza SA, Jhaveri KS. Imaging in male infertility. Radiol Clin. 2012;50(6):1183-200.
12. Jung DC, Park SY, Lee JY. Penile Doppler ultrasonography revisited. Ultrasonography. 2018;37(1):16-24.

Surgical Management of Male Infertility

Manasi Kamalakar Deoghare, JB Sharma

■ INTRODUCTION

Infertility is defined as inability to conceive after 1 year of regular, unprotected intercourse and affects 15% of all couples.[1] In those couples, approximately half are due entirely to the female factor, 20% due to the male factor, and the remaining 30% involving a combination of both.[2] Hence for all infertile couples, a thorough evaluation of both partners is required.

Evaluation of male partner begins with history focusing on age, occupation, diet, smoking, etc. and most importantly semen analysis. All those with abnormal semen analysis parameters are further evaluated. Hormonal evaluation including follicle-stimulating hormone (FSH) and testosterone should be done for infertile men with impaired libido, erectile dysfunction, oligozoospermia or azoospermia, atrophic testes, or evidence of hormonal abnormality on physical evaluation. Azoospermic men should be clinically evaluated to differentiate genital tract obstruction from impaired sperm production initially based on semen volume, physical examination, and FSH levels. Karyotype and Y-chromosome microdeletion analysis should be recommended for men with primary infertility and azoospermia or severe oligozoospermia.[3]

Surgeries for male infertility are divided into four major categories: (1) Diagnostic surgery, (2) surgery to improve sperm production, (3) surgery to improve sperm delivery, and (4) surgery to retrieve sperm for use with in vitro fertilization and intracytoplasmic sperm injection (IVF–ICSI).

■ DIAGNOSTIC SURGERY[4]

In the evaluation of the azoospermic male, it is important to know whether spermatogenesis is occurring in the testes and to what degree. Unfortunately, noninvasive tests cannot predict which azoospermic men will actually harbor sperm within the testicle. The histological or cytological identification of mature spermatozoa within sampled testicular tissue is the only reliable predictor of spermatogenesis.[5] In general, testicular tissue may be sampled for diagnostic purposes via two distinct methods—multisite fine needle aspiration (FNA) (or "testicular mapping") and open testicular biopsy.

When nonobstructive azoospermia (NOA) is suspected or the clinical picture is unclear, a diagnostic biopsy or fine needle biopsy (FNA) is generally warranted. In some circumstances, a testicular biopsy may be both diagnostic and therapeutic, whereby a biopsy segment, if found to have mature spermatozoa, may be cryopreserved for future use with assisted reproductive technology (ART).

■ SURGERY TO IMPROVE SPERM PRODUCTION

Varicocele is considered to be one of the most common correctable causes of male infertility, occurring in up to 40% of evaluated men.[6]

In varicocele, there is impairment of the normal function of the venous (pampiniform) plexus that drains blood from the testicles. This leads to gravitational pooling of venous blood with concomitant loss of normal testicular temperature regulation and thus affects spermatogenesis.

In men with infertility and palpable varicoceles, varicocelectomy is recommended and it should not be done if varicocele is not palpable and diagnosed solely on the basis of imaging.[7] After varicocelectomy, there is improvement in semen parameters, especially motility and morphology.[8]

The goal of varicocele repair is to ligate or thrombose veins which are contributing to the varices as well as others that have a potential to cause varices in the future, while preserving adequate venous drainage, arteries, vas, and lymphatics. It can be performed by retroperitoneal and laparoscopic approach. Inguinal and subinguinal approaches are now the preferred techniques. A surgical microscope is utilized to identify, isolate, and ligate individual varices so that there is clear visualization of all the structures, thus decreasing complications such as hydrocele formation, varicocele recurrence, and testicular artery injury.[9]

■ SURGERY TO IMPROVE SPERM DELIVERY

After vasectomy, around 6% men desire reversal.[10] For a man who desires restoration of the fertility after vasectomy, there are two options for having a biologic child: Vasectomy reversal or sperm extraction with IVF-ICSI. As first described by Silber,[11] microscopic vasal anastomosis has become preferred technique to achieve a high rate of success. Besides the technical skills of the surgeon, the interval since vasectomy is a key factor in the success of vasectomy reversal. Vasovasotomy is the surgical anastomosis of testicular and abdominal ends of the severed vas. Microsurgical repair shows significantly better results than macroscopic anastomosis. During vasal isolation, an adequate length of vas on both sides is required for a tension-free anastomosis. Surrounding adventitia should be preserved to minimize ischemia and subsequent occlusion. Precise approximation of the lumens is required to achieve the best patency results and minimize sperm leak and granuloma formation. Suturing is generally performed with a double-arm 10-0 for luminal stitches and 9-0 nylon for the seromuscular layer. Vasoepididymostomy can also be performed.

Ejaculatory duct obstruction (EDO): 1–5% of male infertility is associated with EDO.[12] Transrectal ultrasound is used as a standard diagnostic modality. Transurethral resection of ejaculatory ducts is the primary treatment for the EDO.

■ SURGERY TO RETRIEVE SPERM

Azoospermia is defined as the absence of spermatozoa in at least two centrifuged samples of ejaculate. It could be because of obstructive azoospermia (OA) or NOA pathology.

Ideal surgical technique for sperm retrieval would retrieve a sufficient number of spermatozoa to fertilize all the available oocytes, with minimal trauma to the testes and could be repeated multiple times in cases of unsuccessful ART cycle.

■ TESTICULAR SPERM ASPIRATION[13]

Testicular sperm aspiration (TESA) may be performed in men in whom spermatogenesis is thought to be unaffected or at least present. It is usually done under local anesthesia. The testis is punctured and negative pressure is exerted on a 20-mL syringe primed with nutrient medium with 20-gauge needle. The needle is moved back and forth four to five times in different directions without removing it from the site of puncture. There are significantly better sperm retrieval rates in men with OA than with NOA.

■ TESTICULAR SPERM EXTRACTION

Testicular sperm extraction (TESE) differs from TESA in that it requires an incision to reach the testicular tissue. Currently, it is the most frequently used technique for sperm extraction in NOA men with a mean sperm recovery rate of 49.5%.[14]

■ MICROTESTICULAR SPERM EXTRACTION

In comparison with conventional TESE, microTESE has a significant learning curve and requires proficiency in microsurgical techniques and a longer operative time. The technique relies upon the magnifying ability of a surgical microscope to allow identification of the individual seminiferous tubules that are engorged with sperm.

■ PERCUTANEOUS EPIDIDYMAL SPERM ASPIRATION[15]

Percutaneous epididymal sperm aspiration (PESA) is the method of choice in men with OA. Epididymal sperm offers the advantage of great maturity and motility relative to testicular sperm, thus improving pregnancy rates. But the problem with this method is that occasionally, insufficient quantity of sperms is obtained.

This technique is similar to TESA. A 10-mL syringe with 23-gauge needle primed with nutrient medium is inserted into the epididymis and 5 mL of negative pressure is applied. The needle should be moved back and forth inside the epididymis. Once fluid is seen just above the needle hub, it is expelled into the tube with sperm nutrient medium and engorged with sperm.

MICROSCOPIC EPIDIDYMAL SPERM ASPIRATION[14]

Microscopic epididymal sperm aspiration (MESA) requires an operating microscope and proficiency in microsurgical skills similar to microTESE. It is ideal for men with unreconstructable causes of OA such as congenital bilateral absence of vas deference. It can also be done in case of multiple prior surgeries and extensive scarring. Relative to PESA, MESA offers the advantage of controlled exposure of the epididymal tubule with the ability to extract far greater quantities of motile sperm. Further, the epididymal tunica may be closed surgically to prevent ongoing sperm leakage once sperm is retrieved.

CONCLUSION

There have been lot of advances in the surgical treatment of male infertility. New diagnostic modalities, tailored treatments, and improved microsurgical techniques now lead to higher patency and pregnancy rates with decreased morbidity.

REFERENCES

1. Greenhall E, Vessey M. The prevalence of subfertility: a review of the current confusion and a report of two new studies. Fertil Steril. 1990;54(6):978-83.
2. Thonneau P, Marchand S, Tallec A, Ferial ML, Ducot B, Lansac J, et al. Incidence and main causes of infertility in a resident population (1,850,000) of three French regions (1988-1989). Hum Reprod Oxf Engl. 1991;6(6):811-6.
3. American Society for Reproductive Medicine. (2020). Diagnosis and treatment of infertility in men: AUA/ASRM guideline part I. [online] Available from https://www.asrm.org/practice-guidance/practice-committee-documents/diagnosis-and-treatment-of-infertility-in-men-auaasrm-guideline-part-i-2020/ [Last accessed April, 2024].
4. Lopushnyan NA, Walsh TJ. Surgical techniques for the management of male infertility. Asian J Androl. 2012;14(1):94-102.
5. Ezeh UI, Taub NA, Moore HD, Cooke ID. Establishment of predictive variables associated with testicular sperm retrieval in men with non-obstructive azoospermia. Hum Reprod Oxf Engl. 1999;14(4):1005-12.

6. Nature Reviews Urology. (2017). Varicocele and male infertility. [online] Available from https://www.nature.com/articles/nrurol.2017.98 [Last accessed April, 2024].
7. American Society for Reproductive Medicine. (2021). Diagnosis and treatment of infertility in men: AUA/ASRM guideline part II. [online] Available from https://www.asrm.org/practice-guidance/practice-committee-documents/diagnosis-and-treatment-of-infertility-in-men-aua-asrm-guideline-part2/ [Last accessed April, 2024].
8. Kibar Y, Seckin B, Erduran D. The effects of subinguinal varicocelectomy on Kruger morphology and semen parameters. J Urol. 2002;168(3):1071-4.
9. Diegidio P, Jhaveri JK, Ghannam S, Pinkhasov R, Shabsigh R, Fisch H. Review of current varicocelectomy techniques and their outcomes. BJU Int. 2011;108(7):1157-72.
10. Brandell RA, Goldstein M. Vasectomy reversal. Compr Ther. 2000;26(1):39-43.
11. Silber SJ. Microsurgery in clinical urology. Urology. 1975;6(2):150-3.
12. Pryor JP, Hendry WF. Ejaculatory duct obstruction in subfertile males: analysis of 87 patients. Fertil Steril. 1991;56(4):725-30.
13. Coward RM, Mills JN. A step-by-step guide to office-based sperm retrieval for obstructive azoospermia. Transl Androl Urol. 2017;6(4):730-44.
14. Donoso P, Tournaye H, Devroey P. Which is the best sperm retrieval technique for non-obstructive azoospermia? A systematic review. Hum Reprod Update. 2007;13(6):539-49.
15. Shah R. Surgical sperm retrieval: Techniques and their indications. Indian J Urol. 2011;27(1):102-9.

Sperm Retrieval Techniques

Sunil Jindal, Anshu Jindal

■ INTRODUCTION

Azoospermia, the absence of sperm in the semen, presents a formidable challenge in the realm of male infertility treatment. Historically, treatment options were limited, often involving reconstructive surgery or donor insemination. However, the landscape changed dramatically with the advent of assisted reproductive technologies (ART), particularly intracytoplasmic sperm injection (ICSI), which revolutionized the management of male infertility.[1]

■ EVOLUTION OF SPERM RETRIEVAL TECHNIQUES

The evolution of sperm retrieval techniques is a testament to the relentless pursuit of solutions for azoospermia. Early pioneers in the field laid the foundation for modern techniques, refining approaches to maximize sperm retrieval rates (SRRs) while minimizing procedural risks.

■ TECHNIQUES FOR SPERM RETRIEVAL FROM THE EPIDIDYMIS

Microsurgical Epididymal Sperm Aspiration

Procedure

Microsurgical epididymal sperm aspiration (MESA) involves meticulous microsurgical dissection of the epididymis using an operating microscope. The surgeon navigates through the epididymal tubules, aspirating sperm from various locations. This technique is particularly effective in cases of obstructive azoospermia.

Success Rates

Numerous studies have reported high success rates with MESA, especially when coupled with advanced ART techniques such as ICSI. Success often depends on the surgeon's skill and the patient's specific anatomy.

Case Study

A 35-year-old male diagnosed with obstructive azoospermia underwent MESA, resulting in the successful retrieval of motile sperm for subsequent ICSI. The couple achieved a successful pregnancy and delivered a healthy baby.

Open Fine Needle Aspiration

Procedure
Open fine needle aspiration (OFNA) offers a less complex alternative to MESA, involving direct puncture of the epididymal ductule using a fine needle. This technique reduces surgical time and resource utilization while maintaining efficacy in sperm retrieval.

Comparative Studies
Comparative studies have shown comparable success rates between OFNA and MESA, highlighting OFNA's role as a viable option in selected cases of obstructive azoospermia.

Percutaneous Epididymal Sperm Aspiration

Procedure
Percutaneous epididymal sperm aspiration (PESA) is a minimally invasive technique performed under local anesthesia. A needle is inserted through the scrotal skin into the epididymis and spermatic fluid is aspirated **(Figs. 1 and 2)**. PESA is often preferred for its simplicity and lower invasiveness compared to microsurgical approaches.

Advantages and Considerations
Percutaneous epididymal sperm aspiration is associated with shorter recovery times and reduced surgical complexity. However, it may have lower SRRs compared to microsurgical techniques in certain cases.

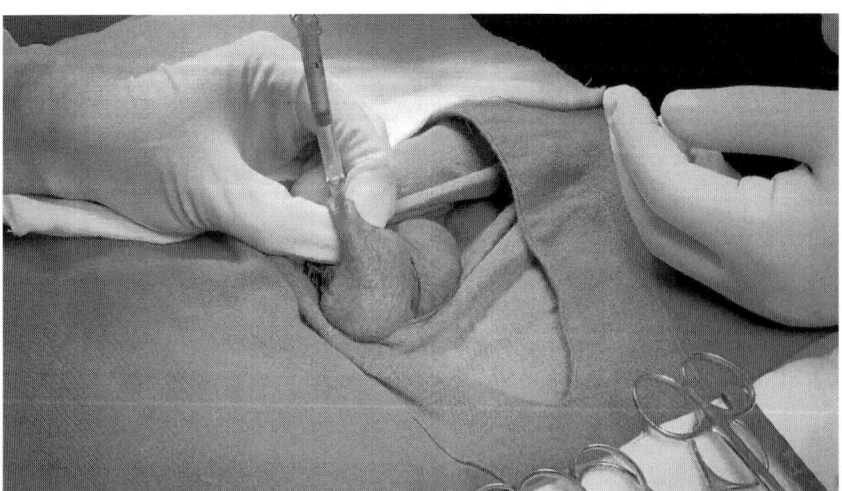

Fig. 1: PESA procedure. *(For color version, see Plate 1).*

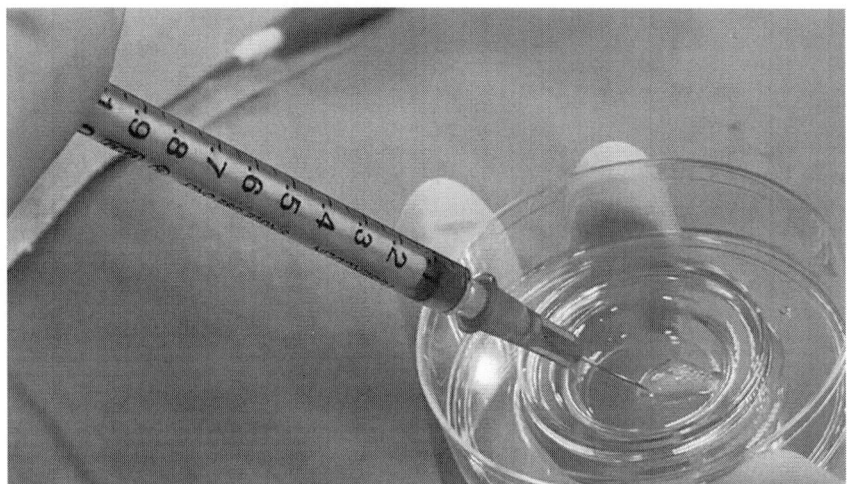

Fig. 2: PESA sample. *(For color version, see Plate 2).*

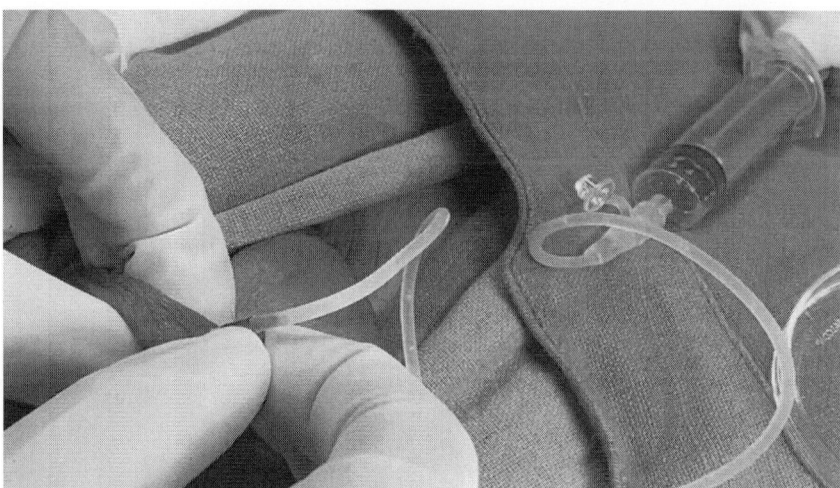

Fig. 3: Testicular sperm aspiration. *(For color version, see Plate 2).*

■ TECHNIQUES FOR SPERM RETRIEVAL FROM THE TESTES

Nonmicrosurgical Approaches

- *Testicular sperm aspiration (TESA)/testicular fine needle aspiration biopsy (FNAB):* Involves using a 20- or 22-G scalp vein needle to aspirate fluid and tiny pieces of testicular tissue for sperm inspection **(Fig. 3)**.
- *Needle aspiration biopsy (NAB)/needle testicular sperm extraction (nTESE):* Utilizes an 18-G scalp vein needle to obtain a core of seminiferous tubules for sperm retrieval. This method is less traumatic than

TESA as it aims to acquire a proper piece of testicular tissue without extensive tissue maceration.

Success Rates and Challenges

While TESA/FNAB can yield viable sperm, success rates may vary depending on testicular histology and spermatogenic capacity. Patients with severe testicular damage or impaired spermatogenesis may have lower success rates.

Emerging Research

Recent studies explore the use of advanced imaging techniques, such as multiparametric ultrasound to improve the accuracy of testicular sperm retrieval and enhance success rates.

Microsurgical Techniques

Procedure

Microsurgical TESE (Micro-TESE) is a sophisticated microsurgical procedure performed under high magnification using an operating microscope. The surgeon meticulously dissects testicular tissue, identifying areas with potential sperm production **(Figs. 4 and 5)**. This targeted approach minimizes tissue damage and maximizes SRRs.

Indications and Success Rates

Micro-TESE is often recommended for men with nonobstructive azoospermia or those with previous failed sperm retrieval attempts. Studies have shown

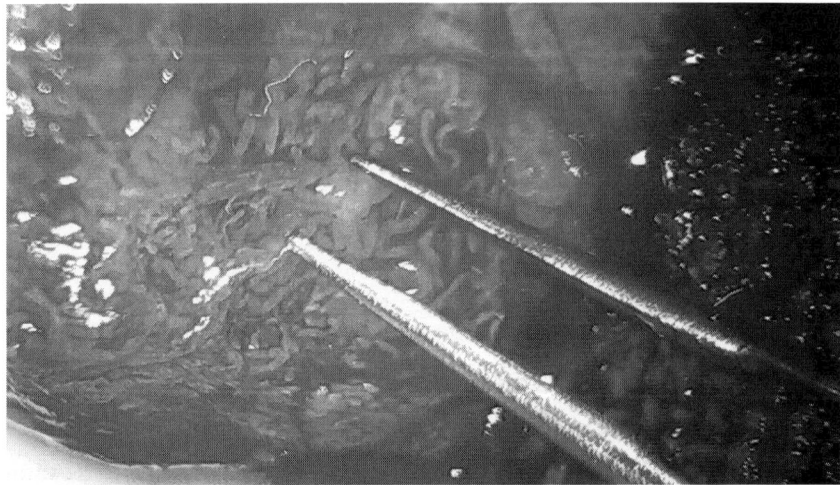

Fig. 4: Micro-TESE in maturation arrest. *(For color version, see Plate 3).*

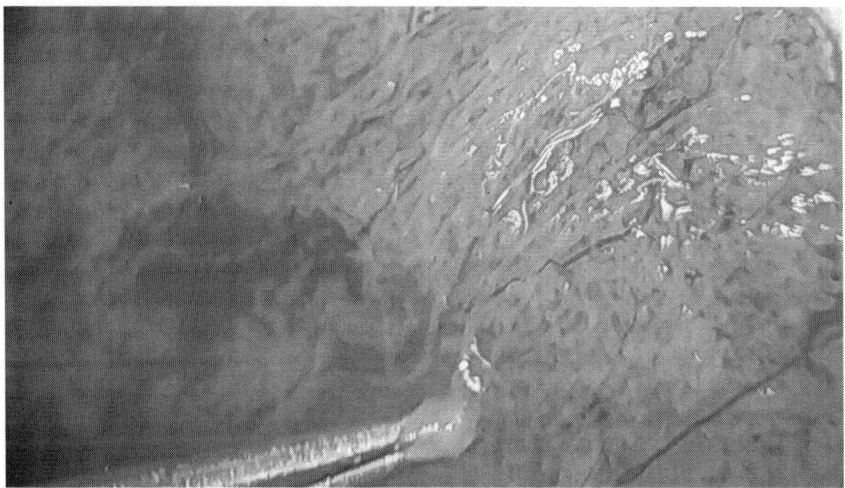

Fig. 5: Micro-TESE in Sertoli only syndrome. *(For color version, see Plate 3).*

significantly higher SRRs with micro-TESE compared to conventional open biopsy techniques.

Case Study

A 30-year-old male with Klinefelter syndrome and nonobstructive azoospermia underwent micro-TESE, resulting in the successful retrieval of viable sperm for ICSI. The couple achieved pregnancy after multiple cycles of ART.

Studies have shown varying success rates in sperm retrieval based on the technique used:
- Micro-TESE has been reported to have the highest SRRs compared to conventional TESE (cTESE) and percutaneous techniques such as TESA.[2]
- Micro-TESE is particularly effective in men with specific conditions like Sertoli cell-only syndrome, although its superiority over cTESE is debated in cases of maturation arrest.
- Complications associated with operative sperm retrieval include infection, bleeding, hematoma, and testicular damage, with micro-TESE causing less physiological damage compared to multiple biopsies by cTESE.[3]

Hybrid Techniques (Single Seminiferous Tubule Mapping)

Procedure

Single seminiferous tubule (SST) mapping involves microsurgical inspection and biopsy of individual seminiferous tubules **(Figs. 6 and 7)**. This precise

Sperm Retrieval Techniques

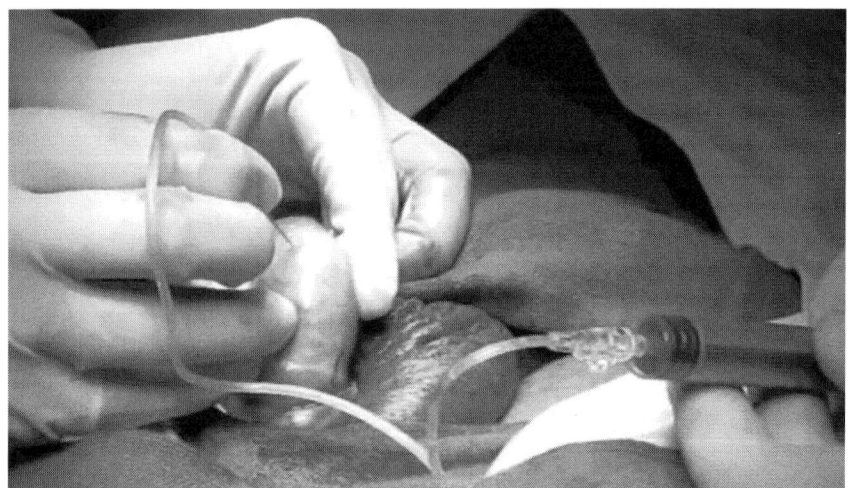

Fig. 6: Needle placement in SST. *(For color version, see Plate 4).*

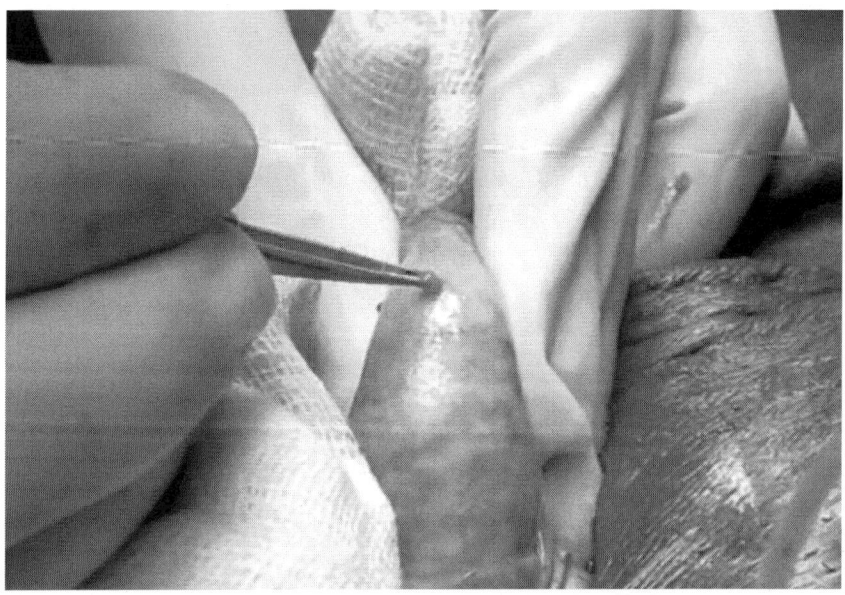

Fig. 7: Core tissue extraction in SST. *(For color version, see Plate 4).*

approach allows for targeted sampling of testicular tissue, increasing the likelihood of sperm retrieval.

Advantages and Applications

Single seminiferous tubule mapping is particularly useful in cases where specific areas of spermatogenesis are preserved within the testes. It minimizes unnecessary tissue trauma and optimizes the use of retrieved sperm for ART procedures.

■ EFFICACY OF SPERM RETRIEVAL

The efficacy of sperm retrieval techniques depends on various factors, including the underlying cause of azoospermia, testicular histology, hormonal levels, genetic factors, and individual patient characteristics. While some techniques, such as micro-TESE, consistently yield high success rates, personalized approaches are essential to optimize outcomes for each patient.

■ COMPLICATIONS AND CONSIDERATIONS

Operative sperm retrieval procedures, including micro-TESE, carry potential risks such as infection, bleeding, hematoma formation, and testicular damage. However, advances in surgical techniques, anesthesia protocols, and postoperative care have significantly reduced the incidence of complications.

■ SPERM RETRIEVAL IN SPECIFIC CONDITIONS

- *Ejaculatory failure:* In cases of ejaculatory dysfunction, such as retrograde ejaculation or anejaculation, testicular sperm retrieval techniques such as NAB are preferred over epididymal techniques due to the absence of obstruction.
- *Necrozoospermia:* Despite immotile or dead sperm in ejaculated samples, viable sperm can often be retrieved from the testis using techniques such as NAB or micro-TESE. The ability to retrieve viable sperm offers hope for fertility restoration in these challenging cases.

■ OPTIMIZING SPERM RETRIEVAL STRATEGIES

Tailored approaches to sperm retrieval consider the unique characteristics of each patient, including the type of azoospermia (obstructive vs. nonobstructive), spermatogenic capacity, previous surgical interventions, hormonal levels, and genetic factors. Multidisciplinary collaboration between andrologists, urologists, reproductive endocrinologists, and embryologists is crucial in developing personalized treatment plans.

■ ADVANCES IN HORMONAL STIMULATION

Hormonal therapies, such as gonadotropin-releasing hormone (GnRH) agonists and human chorionic gonadotropin (hCG), play a role in optimizing spermatogenesis before sperm retrieval procedures. These hormonal interventions are especially beneficial in cases of hypogonadotropic hypogonadism and secondary infertility. This is yet to be proven by more robust studies.[4]

■ ULTRASOUND-GUIDED TECHNIQUES

The integration of ultrasound guidance into sperm retrieval procedures has significantly enhanced precision and safety. Ultrasound imaging helps identify optimal biopsy sites, avoid vascular structures, and reduce the risk of complications such as hematoma formation.

■ PREDICTORS OF SUCCESSFUL SPERM RETRIEVAL

There are conflicting reports on predictors of sperm retrieval success as follows:
- Some studies suggest lower SRRs with high follicle-stimulating hormone (FSH) levels and small testes, while others find no correlation.
- Testicular histology, hormonal levels, and genetic factors may influence the success of sperm retrieval, but no single parameter can predict sperm presence with 100% accuracy.

■ CLINICAL CONSIDERATIONS AND DECISION-MAKING

Clinical decision-making in sperm retrieval involves a comprehensive evaluation of the patient's medical history, diagnostic test results, testicular histology, hormonal profile, genetic factors, and previous fertility treatments. Key considerations include:
- *Type of azoospermia:* Distinguishing between obstructive and nonobstructive azoospermia guides the selection of appropriate sperm retrieval techniques. Obstructive azoospermia often necessitates epididymal sperm retrieval methods, while nonobstructive azoospermia may require testicular sperm extraction techniques.
- *Spermatogenic capacity:* Assessing the patient's spermatogenic capacity through testicular histology, hormonal levels, and genetic testing helps predict the likelihood of successful sperm retrieval.
- *Previous surgical interventions:* Patients with a history of prior scrotal surgeries, testicular trauma, or failed sperm retrieval attempts require careful consideration and may benefit from advanced microsurgical techniques.
- *Testicular histology:* Testicular biopsy findings, such as the presence of spermatogenesis, germ cell maturation, and the extent of testicular damage, influence the choice of sperm retrieval approach.
- *Hormonal status:* Hormonal evaluation, including FSH, luteinizing hormone (LH), testosterone, and estradiol levels, provides insights into testicular function and spermatogenic potential.

- *Genetic factors:* Genetic testing for chromosomal abnormalities, Y-chromosome microdeletions, and specific gene mutations helps identify genetic causes of male infertility and informs treatment strategies.

■ FUTURE DIRECTIONS AND INNOVATIONS

The field of sperm retrieval continues to evolve, driven by ongoing research and technological advancements. Key areas of focus for future innovations include:
- *Genetic and molecular insights:* Advancements in genetic testing, genomic sequencing, and molecular diagnostics offer deeper insights into the genetic basis of male infertility. Targeted therapies based on genetic findings may enhance treatment outcomes.
- *Pharmacological interventions:* Continued research on novel pharmacological agents, including selective androgen receptor modulators (SARMs), gonadotropin analogs, and antioxidants, aims to improve spermatogenesis and sperm quality.
- *Stem cell therapy:* Emerging strategies in stem cell therapy, including the use of mesenchymal stem cells (MSCs), spermatogonial stem cells (SSCs), and induced pluripotent stem cells (iPSCs), hold promise for regenerating testicular tissue and restoring fertility.
- *Artificial intelligence (AI) and machine learning (ML):* Integration of AI algorithms, deep learning models, and image analysis techniques into sperm retrieval procedures enhance procedural accuracy, automate sperm identification, and predict optimal biopsy sites.
- *Nanotechnology and biomaterials:* Advancements in nanotechnology, microfluidics, and biomaterial engineering lead to the development of advanced sperm-sorting devices, microsurgical tools, and drug delivery systems, optimizing sperm quality and reproductive outcomes.

■ ETHICAL CONSIDERATIONS AND PATIENT COUNSELING

Ethical considerations in sperm retrieval encompass informed consent, patient autonomy, confidentiality, genetic counseling, and reproductive rights. Key ethical principles include:
- *Informed consent:* Patients undergoing sperm retrieval procedures must receive comprehensive information about the risks, benefits, alternatives, and potential outcomes of the procedure. Informed consent ensures patient understanding and voluntary participation in fertility treatments.
- *Genetic counseling:* It plays a crucial role in educating patients about genetic testing, hereditary conditions, inheritance risks, and family planning options. It empowers patients to make informed decisions about genetic screening, preimplantation genetic testing (PGT), and gamete donation.

- *Reproductive rights:* Patients have the right to make autonomous decisions regarding their reproductive health, including fertility preservation, embryo disposition, and family-building options. Respect for patient autonomy and reproductive choices is fundamental in ethical fertility care.
- *Confidentiality and privacy:* Maintaining patient confidentiality, data privacy, and medical records security is essential in protecting patient rights and fostering trust between healthcare providers and patients.
- *Equity and access:* Ensuring equitable access to fertility services, regardless of socioeconomic status, geographic location, or demographic factors promotes fairness, inclusivity, and healthcare equity in reproductive medicine.

GLOBAL COLLABORATION AND DATA SHARING

Global collaboration, data sharing, and knowledge exchange among fertility experts, research institutions, regulatory agencies, and patient advocacy groups drive innovation, standardization, and quality improvement in sperm retrieval techniques. Initiatives like Global Andrology Forum or GAF which has initiated a movement across all continents and all major countries by involving their top scientists to collaborate on these initiatives.

CONCLUSION

The evolution of sperm retrieval techniques reflects a dynamic interplay between scientific advancements, clinical expertise, ethical considerations, and patient-centered care in male infertility management. From traditional approaches like PESA to micro-TESE to cutting-edge innovations in stem cell therapy, AI-driven diagnostics, and nanotechnology, the field continues to evolve, offering new hope and possibilities for individuals and couples on their journey to parenthood.

REFERENCES

1. Shah R. Surgical sperm retrieval: techniques and their indications. Indian J Urol. 2011;27(1):102-9.
2. Punjani N, Kang C, Schlegel PN. Two decades from the introduction of microdissection testicular sperm extraction: how this surgical technique has improved the management of NOA. J Clin Med. 2021;10(7):1374.
3. Esteves SC. Microdissection TESE versus conventional TESE for men with nonobstructive azoospermia undergoing sperm retrieval. Int Braz J Urol. 2022;48(3):569-78.
4. Tharakan T, Corona G, Foran D, Salonia A, Sofikitis N, Giwercman A, et al. Does hormonal therapy improve sperm retrieval rates in men with non-obstructive azoospermia: a systematic review and meta-analysis. Hum Reprod Update. 2022;28(5):609-28.

CHAPTER 7: Medical Management and Nutraceuticals

Pratik Tambe, Suyesha Khanijao

■ INTRODUCTION

Nutraceuticals, a term derived from "nutrition" and "pharmaceuticals", refers to food or food products that provide health and medical benefits, including the prevention and treatment of diseases. Male infertility is a condition characterized by the inability of a man to father a child which is a significant public health issue affecting approximately 7% of men worldwide. Male factor infertility may be due to issues such as low sperm count, poor sperm motility, or abnormal sperm morphology.

Nutraceuticals have gained attention as potential interventions for male infertility due to their ability to modulate various physiological processes that influence reproductive health. We explore the relationship between nutraceuticals and male infertility, including the potential mechanisms of action and evidence supporting their use.

■ NUTRACEUTICALS

Nutraceuticals are used as ingredients of dietary supplements (DS), widely marketed for the prevention or treatment of the most disparate pathological conditions. In 1989, the word "nutraceutical" was coined by Dr Stephen DeFelice who defined it as food or part of food that aids the prevention and/or treatment of diseases and/or disorders. In recent years, due to more and upgraded knowledge about this concept it has gained a lot of popularity in developed countries as an option to improve various aspects of health.

Nutraceuticals are bioactive compounds derived from natural sources that are purported to have beneficial effects on health. These compounds include vitamins, minerals, amino acids, antioxidants, and herbal extracts. In the context of infertility, nutraceuticals are believed to exert their effects by improving reproductive function, balancing hormones, reducing oxidative stress, and enhancing overall health and well-being.[1,2]

■ NUTRACEUTICALS AND MALE REPRODUCTIVE HEALTH

Male infertility can result from various factors including hormonal imbalances, sperm abnormalities, and reproductive tract obstructions. Nutraceuticals have been investigated for their potential to improve male reproductive health by targeting these underlying factors. Several

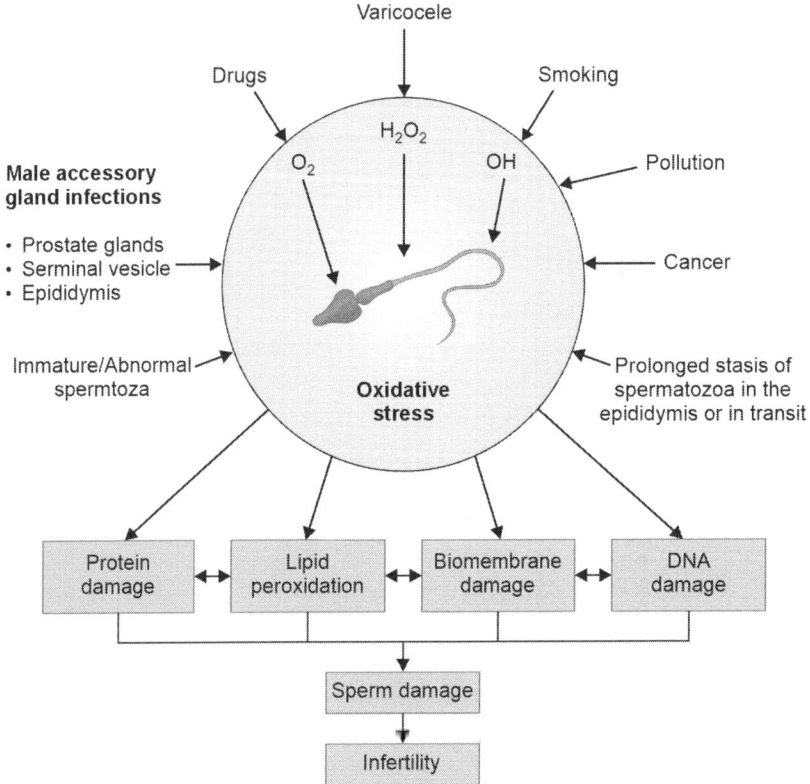

Fig. 1: Reactive oxygen species, impaired sperm function, and male infertility. (DNA: deoxyribonucleic acid)

nutraceutical compounds, such as antioxidants, vitamins, minerals, and herbal extracts, have been studied for their effects on sperm quality, hormone levels, and overall reproductive function.

Antioxidants such as vitamin C, vitamin E, and coenzyme Q10 (CoQ10) are among the most widely studied nutraceuticals in the context of male infertility. These compounds are known for their ability to neutralize reactive oxygen species (ROS) and reduce oxidative stress, which can damage sperm deoxyribonucleic acid (DNA) and impair sperm function. By reducing oxidative stress, antioxidants may improve sperm motility, morphology, and overall quality, thereby enhancing male fertility **(Fig. 1)**.

In addition to antioxidants, certain vitamins and minerals play essential roles in male reproductive function. For example, vitamin D has been associated with testosterone production and sperm quality, while zinc is crucial for sperm development and motility. Nutraceuticals containing these nutrients may support male fertility by addressing potential deficiencies and optimizing reproductive hormone levels.

Furthermore, herbal extracts and phytochemicals have been investigated for their potential effects on male infertility. For instance, *Tribulus terrestris*, a plant extract, has been traditionally used to enhance male fertility and libido. Research suggests that it may exert beneficial effects on sperm parameters and reproductive hormone levels, although further studies are needed to confirm its efficacy.

■ MECHANISMS OF ACTION

The mechanisms through which nutraceuticals exert their effects on male infertility are diverse and multifaceted. One of the primary mechanisms involves the modulation of oxidative stress and inflammation. Oxidative stress, characterized by an imbalance between ROS production and antioxidant defenses, can impair sperm function and contribute to male infertility. Nutraceutical antioxidants help restore this balance, thereby protecting sperm from oxidative damage and preserving their viability and fertility potential.

Moreover, nutraceuticals may influence male reproductive health by regulating hormone levels and signaling pathways. For example, certain compounds may enhance testosterone production, improve sperm maturation, or modulate the expression of genes involved in spermatogenesis. By targeting these pathways, nutraceuticals can support the overall function of the male reproductive system and mitigate factors contributing to infertility.

■ SCIENTIFIC EVIDENCE AND CLINICAL STUDIES

Numerous clinical studies have investigated the effects of nutraceuticals on male infertility, providing valuable insights into their potential efficacy. Systematic reviews and meta-analyses which evaluated the impact of antioxidant supplementation on male infertility have concluded that antioxidant therapy is associated with significant improvements in sperm concentration, motility, and morphology, highlighting the potential of nutraceutical antioxidants as adjunct treatments for male infertility.

Similarly, clinical trials which examined the effects of specific nutraceutical compounds, such as CoQ10 and carnitine on sperm parameters and reproductive outcomes have reported promising results, indicating that nutraceutical supplementation may enhance sperm quality and pregnancy rates in couples undergoing fertility treatment.

Furthermore, emerging research is now exploring the synergistic effects of combining multiple nutraceuticals to target different aspects of male reproductive health. By formulating comprehensive nutraceutical blends, researchers aim to optimize the therapeutic potential and address the multifactorial nature of male infertility. We now address the individual molecules with their supporting evidence which is currently available.

COENZYME Q10

This is a naturally occurring antioxidant in the body that supports metabolism and protects cells from free radicals. It works by combating oxidation and protecting sperm from damage, thus helps improve seminal parameters (count and motility).

Studies have shown that CoQ10 supplementation may improve sperm quality and motility in men with infertility. It may help in reducing oxidative stress and enhance sperm motility and DNA integrity. It also decreases the follicle-stimulating hormone (FSH) and increases inhibin, thereby having a positive effect on testicular function and improving spermatogenesis **(Fig. 2)**.

The recommended dosage is 300 mg/day for 3–6 months and improvements in semen parameters begin after 3–6 months of treatment but disappear when supplementation is discontinued. Further studies are needed to establish the optimal CoQ10 dosage and the possible superiority of coadministration with other molecules compared to monotherapy.

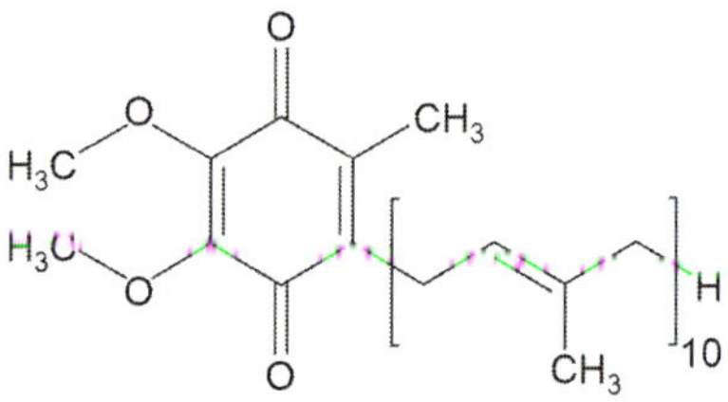

Fig. 2: Chemical structure of coenzyme Q10.

A meta-analysis in 2020 showed significant improvement in sperm concentration and motility. The fundamental role CoQ10 plays in male fertility and the redox state is proven by the direct correlation between sperm count, ubiquinol, and the inverse correlation between hydroperoxide-ubiquinol, respectively.[3,4]

CARNITINES

Carnitines, also known as l-carnitine or by its active form, l-acetylcarnitine, play an essential role in bioenergy production by functioning as a long-chain fatty acid transporter in the mitochondria. It protects cell membranes and exerts antiapoptotic actions. They are highly abundant in the epididymis, where they are constantly secreted **(Fig. 3)**.

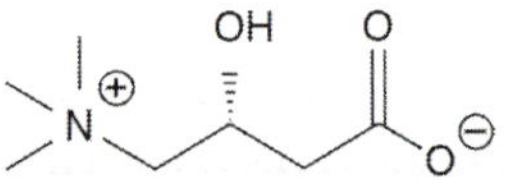

Fig. 3: Chemical structure of l-carnitine.

A direct relation between carnitines and sperm motility has been proven in several clinical trials. The supplemented dosages of l-carnitine range from 2 to 3 g/day. A positive correlation between seminal l-carnitine and sperm count levels, motility, and morphology have been proven by recent studies.[5,6]

LYCOPENE

Lycopene is a naturally occurring, primary carotenoid found in the human body. High concentrations of lycopene are found in the human testes. It does not have vitamin A activity as it lacks a beta-ionic ring. It is a potent antioxidant which exhibits antiproliferative, immunomodulatory, anti-inflammatory effects, and promotes cell differentiation (**Fig. 4**).

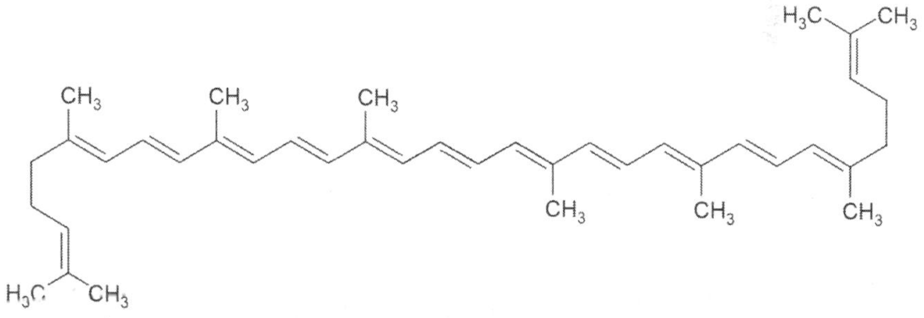

Fig. 4: Chemical structure of lycopene.

Lycopene supplementation 25 mg/day for 12 weeks has proven to improve sperm count and concentration in a recent randomized controlled trial (RCT). Lycopene supplementation 10 mg twice daily for 3 months found that seven couples spontaneously conceived during the 3-month period before even undergoing in vitro fertilization (IVF).[7,8]

VITAMINS C, E, AND D

Vitamin C or ascorbic acid is capable of reducing metals and regenerating vitamin E from its oxidized form. Humans cannot synthesize it and it needs to be supplemented in diet or via nutraceutical administration. It prevents agglutination and protects against DNA damage caused by ROS. A clinical trial involving overweight and obese men supplemented with vitamin C demonstrated improved semen concentration and motility. A prospective cohort demonstrated a positive relationship between vitamin C intake and fertilization rates in couples undergoing ART.[9,10]

Vitamin E is a lipid-soluble antioxidant which protects cell membranes and prevents lipid peroxidation. It cannot be synthesized in humans and requires dietary supplementation. It is essential for testosterone biosynthesis and modulation of telomerase activity. Vitamin E supplementation of

200 mg/day for 3 months improves lipid peroxidation activity and improved fertilization rates as well.[11,12]

Vitamin D is important for reproductive health, as it influences hormone production and immune function. Low levels of vitamin D have been linked to infertility in both men and women. It has an important role in the production of sperm cells.

Low levels of vitamin D have been associated with decreased sperm count and motility and to lower levels of testosterone. Supplementation may improve sperm morphology and reduce DNA damage in sperm cells. Vitamin D maintains various hormones including inhibin B which is found to be lower in men with vitamin D deficiency. Inhibin B is a quantitative marker of normal spermatogenesis.

■ FOLIC ACID

Vitamin B_9 or folic acid is a water-soluble compound essential in DNA metabolism. It is required for the synthesis of uracil to thymine, protecting against mutations and DNA strand breaks. DNA methylation and gene expression are regulated by this vitamin, preventing abnormal chromosomal replication and mitochondrial DNA deletions. Supplementation is known to increase sperm concentration but not motility and morphology.[13]

■ ZINC

Zinc has reducing properties and plays a role in signaling, enzymatic activities, regulation of normal growth, sexual maturation, and decreasing mitochondrial oxidative stress. Zinc also has an important role in human sperm motility and acrosome reaction. It serves to protect against sperm decondensation, aids sperm motility, membrane stabilization, and antioxidant capacity. Groups supplemented with zinc sulfate exhibit a higher conception rate (22.5%) compared to placebo (4.2%).[14,15]

■ SELENIUM

Selenium improves semen parameters such as total sperm count, progressive motility, total motility, and normal morphology. Higher clinical pregnancy rates and live births are also associated with higher seminal selenium levels.[16]

■ L-ARGININE

Required for the synthesis of proteins and gets converted to nitric oxide (NO) in the body. NO helps blood vessels to relax which helps more oxygen-rich blood to circulate through arteries. Healthy blood flow to the arteries of the penis is essential for normal erectile function. Arginine plays an important role in sperm production and motility. Research shows supplementation may improve sperm count and quality. It also performs an essential role in spermatogenesis. The typical dose for supplementation ranges from 2 to 4 g/day **(Fig. 5)**.

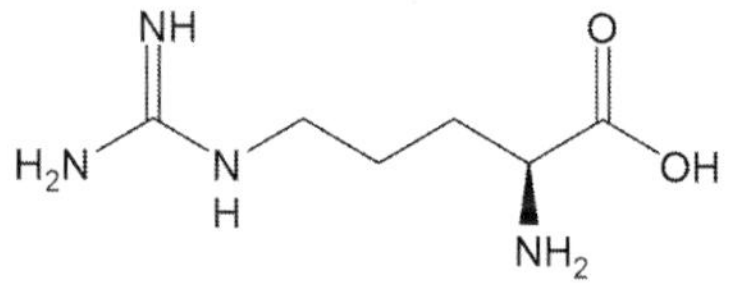

Fig. 5: Chemical structure of L-arginine.

N-ACETYL CYSTEINE

Originally used as a mucolytic, it is a powerful antioxidant. Multiple studies have shown benefits vis-à-vis male infertility. N-acetyl cysteine (NAC) reduces apoptotic rates in testicular cells by 68%. Sperm parameters proven to improve are volume, motility, count, concentration, and normal morphology. It may also help to counteract sperm viscosity, liquefaction time, and DNA fragmentation **(Fig. 6)**.[17]

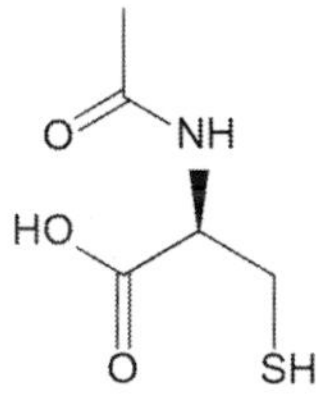

Fig. 6: Chemical structure of N-acetyl cysteine.

MELATONIN

It is secreted by the pineal gland and is proven to occur in higher concentrations in fertile men. It has been shown to decrease DNA fragmentation and increase sperm viability. A systematic review and meta-analysis about melatonin and assisted reproductive technology (ART) concluded that melatonin enriched cultures yield higher quality embryos **(Fig. 7)**.[18]

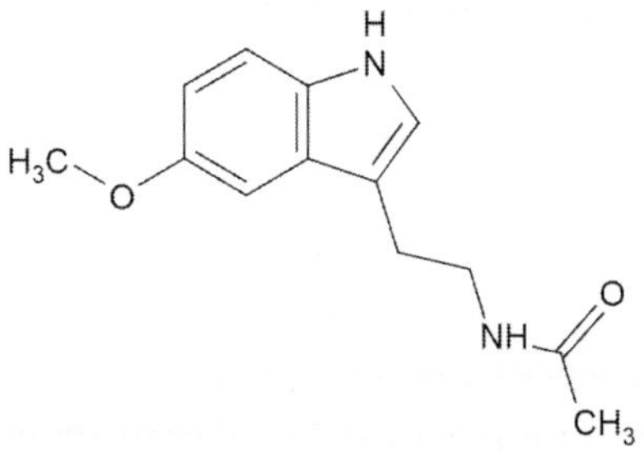

Fig. 7: Chemical structure of melatonin.

OMEGA-3 FATTY ACIDS

These are precursors to eicosanoids and have anti-inflammatory and antioxidant properties. The testes and spermatozoa have a higher concentration of polyunsaturated fatty acids and effective fertilization depends on the lipid composition of the sperm membrane. Omega-3 fatty acids positively affect the concentration, morphology, and functioning of sperm. It is also known that eicosapentaenoic acid (EPA) and/or docosahexaenoic acid (DHA) supplementation with fatty acids significantly increases sperm motility and DHA concentration in semen.[19,20]

GLUTATHIONE

This is one of the most abundant endogenous antioxidants found in the body and plays an important role in maintaining exogenous antioxidants (i.e., vitamins C and E) in their active reduced roles. It is produced in the liver and synthesized from cysteine, glutamic acid, and glycine **(Fig. 8)**.

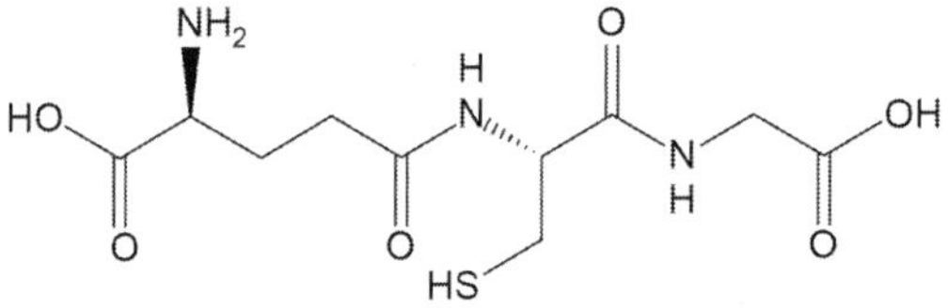

Fig. 8: Chemical structure of glutathione.

Glutathione supplementation in infertile men has been demonstrated to improve sperm motility. Men with varicoceles have a 10% increase in total sperm motility over baseline with treatment ($p < 0.01$). Supplementation in combination with vitamins C and E has also been associated with improved sperm count and decreased DNA fragmentation. Supplementation up to 3 g has been demonstrated to be safe. Regular intake of glutathione-rich foods, whey protein, as well as biochemical precursors, such as (NAC or α-lipoic acid, can maintain normal physiological concentrations for antioxidant benefits.

UPDATED SYSTEMATIC REVIEW AND NETWORK META-ANALYSIS 2023

This most recent systematic review included 64 studies with 94 individual study arms. It is the first of its kind to compare all dietary interventions in a single study. Meta-regression identified that improvement in the sperm count, motility, and morphology translated into increased pregnancy rates ($p < 0.001$; $p < 0.001$; $p < 0.002$, respectively).

Significantly, l-carnitine with micronutrient therapy [risk ratio (RR): 3.60, 95% confidence interval (CI) 1.86, 6.98, $p = 0.0002$], followed by zinc

(RR 5.39, 95% CI 1.26, 23.04, $p = 0.02$), significantly improved pregnancy rates. Men with oligozoospermia (RR 4.89), followed by oligoasthenozoospermia (RR 4.20) and asthenoteratozoospermia (RR 3.53), showed a significant increase in pregnancy rates.[21]

CONCLUSION

Nutraceuticals represent a promising avenue for addressing male infertility through their ability to modulate oxidative stress, hormone levels, and reproductive function. Antioxidants, vitamins, minerals, and herbal extracts are among the key nutraceuticals studied in the context of male reproductive health with evidence supporting their potential benefits for sperm quality and fertility outcomes.

While further research is needed to elucidate the optimal formulations and dosages of nutraceutical interventions, the existing evidence underscores the potential of nutraceuticals as adjunctive therapies for male infertility. As our understanding of the intricate interplay between nutraceuticals and male reproductive health continues to evolve, these interventions may offer new opportunities for improving fertility outcomes and addressing the global burden of male infertility.

REFERENCES

1. Garolla A, Petre GC, Francini-Pessenti F, de Toni L, Vitagliano A, Nisio AD, et al. Dietary supplements for male infertility: a critical evaluation of their composition. Nutrients. 2020;12(5):1472.
2. De Rose AF, Baldi M, Gallo F, Rossi P, Gattuccio I, Marino A, et al. The management of male infertility: from nutraceuticals to diagnostics. Int J Med Device Adjuv Treat. 2018;1(1):e110.
3. Vishvkarma R, Alahmar AT, Gupta G, Rajender S. Coenzyme Q10 Effect on Semen Parameters: Profound or Meagre? Andrologia. 2020;52:e13570.
4. Balercia G, Mancini A, Paggi F, Tiano L, Pontecorvi A, Boscaro M, et al. Coenzyme Q10 and Male Infertility. J Endocrinol Investig. 2009;32:626-32.
5. Torres-Arce E, Vizmanos B, Babio N, Márquez-Sandoval F, Salas-Huetos A. Dietary antioxidants in the treatment of male infertility: counteracting oxidative stress. Biology (Basel). 2021;10(3):241.
6. Martínez-Holguín E, Lledó-García E, Rebollo-Román Á, González-García J. Antioxidants to improve sperm quality. In: Aitken J, Mortimer D, Kovacs G (Eds). Male and Sperm Factors that Maximize IVF Success. Cambridge, UK: Cambridge University Press; 2020. pp. 106-120.
7. Nouri M, Amani R, Nasr-Esfahani M, Tarrahi MJ. The effects of lycopene supplement on the spermatogram and seminal oxidative stress in infertile men: a randomized, double-blind, placebo-controlled clinical trial. Phytother Res. 2019;33:3203-11.
8. Filipcikova R, Oborna I, Brezinova J, Novotny J, Wojewodka G, De Sanctis JB, et al. Lycopene improves the distorted ratio between AA/DHA in the seminal

plasma of infertile males and increases the likelihood of successful pregnancy. Biomed Pap Med Fac Univ Palacky Olomouc Czech Repub. 2015;159:077-082.
9. Rafiee B, Morowvat MH, Rahimi-Ghalati N. Comparing the Effectiveness of dietary vitamin C and exercise interventions on fertility parameters in normal obese men. Urol J. 2016;13:2635-9.
10. Li MC, Chiu YH, Gaskins AJ, Mínguez-Alarcón L, Nassan FL, Williams PL, et al. Men's intake of vitamin C and β-carotene is positively related to fertilization rate but not to live birth rate in couples undergoing infertility treatment. J Nutr. 2019;149:1977-84.
11. Geva E, Bartoov B, Zabludovsky N, Lessing JB, Lerner-Geva L, Amit A. The effect of antioxidant treatment on human spermatozoa and fertilization rate in an in vitro fertilization program. Fertil Steril. 1996;66:430-4.
12. Suleiman SA, Ali ME, Zaki ZM, el-Malik EM, Nasr MA. Lipid peroxidation and human sperm motility: protective role of vitamin E. J Androl. 1996;17:530-7.
13. Irani M, Amirian M, Sadeghi R, Lez JL, Roudsari RL. The effect of folate and folate plus zinc supplementation on endocrine parameters and sperm characteristics in sub-fertile men: a systematic review and meta-analysis. Urol J. 2017;14:4069-8.
14. Kerns K, Zigo M, Sutovsky P. Zinc: a necessary ion for mammalian sperm fertilization competency. Int J Mol Sci. 2018;19:4097.
15. Omu AE, Dashti H, Al-Othman S. Treatment of asthenozoospermia with zinc sulphate: andrological, immunological and obstetric outcome. Eur J Obstet Gynecol Reprod Biol. 1998;79:179-84.
16. Wu S, Wang M, Deng Y, Qiu J, Zhang X, Tan J. Associations of toxic and essential trace elements in serum, follicular fluid, and seminal plasma with in vitro fertilization outcomes. Ecotoxicol Environ Saf. 2020;204:110965.
17. Salas-Huetos A, Rosique-Esteban N, Becerra-Tomás N, Vizmanos B, Bulló M, Salas-Salvadó J. The effect of nutrients and dietary supplements on sperm quality parameters: a systematic review and meta-analysis of randomized clinical trials. Adv Nutr. 2018;9:833-48.
18. Hu KL, Ye X, Wang S, Zhang D. Melatonin application in assisted reproductive technology: a systematic review and meta-analysis of randomized trials. Front Endocrinol. 2020;11:160.
19. Skoracka K, Eder P, Łykowska-Szuber L, Dobrowolska A, Krela-Kaźmierczak I. Diet and nutritional factors in male (In)fertility-underestimated factors. J Clin Med. 2020;9(5):1400.
20. Falsig AL, Gleerup CS, Knudsen UB. The influence of omega-3 fatty acids on semen quality markers: A systematic PRISMA review. Andrology. 2019;7:794-803.
21. Zafar MI, Mills KE, Baird CD, Jiang H, Li H. Effectiveness of nutritional therapies in male factor infertility treatment: a systematic review and network meta-analysis. Drugs. 2023;83(6):531-46.

CHAPTER 8: Fertility Preservation in Men

Madhuri Patil

■ INTRODUCTION

Oncofertility is balancing life-preserving treatments with fertility-preserving options. Today, several advances in the management of cancer with innovative technologies are bringing new promises for life after cancer and other life-threatening diseases. But many of these life-saving therapies may also compromise patients' reproductive health and so some intervention is needed to spare fertility.

There are several concerns in the mind of a cancer patient that preclude them from thinking about fertility preservation (FP). These concerns could be as follows:
- They may be overwhelmed by and focused exclusively on the cancer diagnosis.[1]
- They may be unaware that potential fertility loss may occur.[1]
- They may be concerned that pursuing FP will delay their treatment, leading to increased morbidity or mortality.[2]

For these reasons, thorough counseling and informed consent is essential before cancer therapy. All healthcare providers (including medical oncologists, radiation oncologists, urologists, hematologists, pediatric oncologists, and surgeons) should address either together or separately the possibility of infertility with patients treated during their reproductive years (or with parents or guardians of children). They should also discuss the FP options available and refer all potential patients to appropriate reproductive specialists.

■ HOW DOES CANCER AND ITS TREATMENT AFFECT FERTILITY IN MALES?

With cancer, there may be endocrine and nutritional alterations that affect sperm parameters. There is an induction of a hypermetabolic state, whereby tumor cells, due to their rapid proliferation and apoptosis, produce large quantities of spermatotoxic metabolites harmful to the sperms.[3] Stress following cancer or its treatment can result in hormonal alterations that have deleterious effects on sperm production and function.[3] Malignancy that involves deficiencies in vitamins, minerals, and trace elements, which play a critical role in the maintenance of spermatogenetic quality can affect the sperm parameters.[3] Tumors may promote an autoimmune response by producing antisperm antibodies, preventing sperm motility, or by releasing cytokines, leading to germ cell and Leydig cell injury. Leukemia can affect the endocrine system and the hormones that regulate spermatogenesis follicle-stimulating hormone (FSH), luteinizing hormone (LH), testosterone (T), and inhibin B, resulting in impairment in spermatogenesis.[4] It also results in an imbalance in testicular cytokines and growth factors, which impairs spermatogenesis by interrupting the proliferation and differentiation of spermatogonial stem cells (SSCs) and increases the apoptosis of spermatogenic cells, leading to infertility.[4] The effect of acute leukemia is more than that of chronic. Fever usually associated with Hodgkin's disease negatively affects semen parameters; moreover, Hodgkin's disease and germ cell tumors produce direct gonadotoxic effects and affect sperm aneuploidy frequency before treatment.[5,6] Cancer treatments, including surgery, radiotherapy (RT), and chemotherapy (CT), can have a transitory as well as a permanent detrimental impact on male fertility. Combination treatment with RT and CT will induce more gonadotoxicity than either modality alone.[7]

Chemotherapy: Chemotherapeutic drugs act by interrupting vital cell processes and arrest the normal cellular proliferation cycle. **Flowchart 1** illustrates the cytotoxic agents according to their gonadotoxicity [American Society of Clinical Oncology (ASCO) guidelines]. Tyrosine kinase inhibitors also result in oligospermia and affect acrosomal reaction and capacitation.

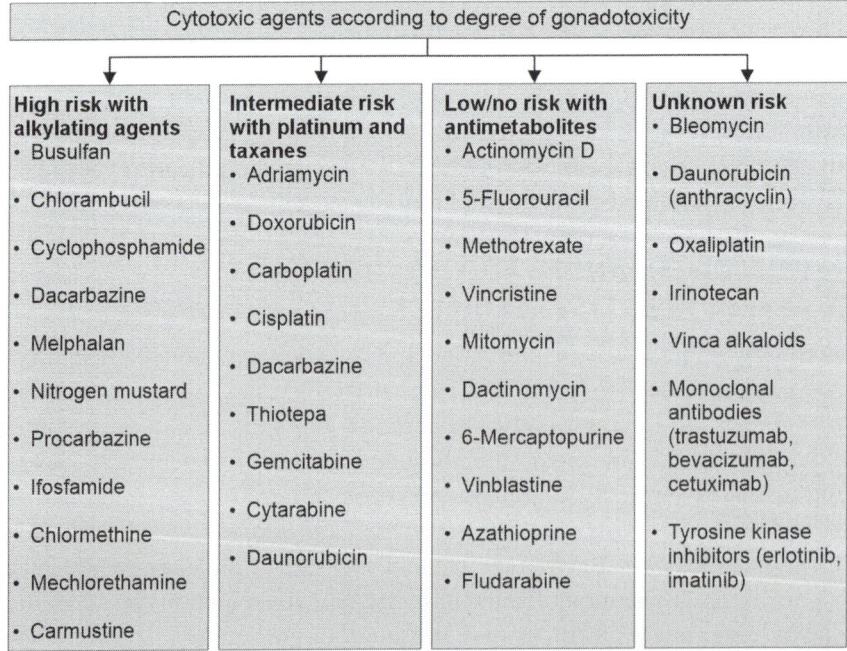

Flowchart 1: Cytotoxic agents according to degree of toxicity.

Flowchart 2: Damage in men with chemotherapeutic agents.

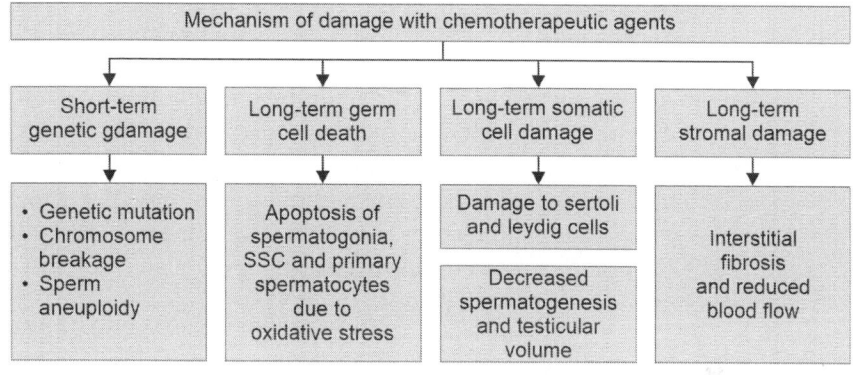

(SSC: spermatogonial stem cell)

Mechanisms of gonadotoxicity of CT in men[8,9] are illustrated in **Flowchart 2**.

Effect of Radiotherapy on Fertility in Men

Type A spermatogonia are classified in the group of the most radiation-sensitive cells as they have a high mitotic rate; on the other hand, Leydig cells are more radioresistant. Transient sterility can be induced after external irradiation by a dose as low as 0.150 Gy to the testis[10] and permanent sterility is to be expected after a dose of 20 Gy in fractionated doses.[11,12] Radiation scatter from RT to pelvic organs can affect testes and repeated irradiation has a cumulative effect.[9] Testosterone production is lowered when Leydig cells are affected.[9] High-dose RT of the pelvis can lead to erectile dysfunction by affecting the pelvic vessels.

Effects of Cranial Irradiation

Effects of cranial irradiation for the treatment of brain tumors may induce infertility by disruption of the hypothalamic–pituitary–gonadal axis and disturbance of gonadotropin secretion. Cranial irradiation in childhood can result in precocious puberty due to cortical disruption and loss of inhibition by the hypothalamus.

Effects of Radioactive Iodine

The dose of radioactive iodine (RAI)[13] used in the treatment of thyroid cancer causes discernible and dose-related germinal epithelium impairment, leading to an increase in FSH. These effects are transient and reverse within a year generally. Radiation dose to testis resulting from RAI treatment for hyperthyroidism may also cause small and transient damage, both to the germinal epithelium and Leydig cells.[14]

Sexual Dysfunction Following Cancer Treatment

Effectively addressing sexual dysfunction can be difficult given the varied etiologies and multifactorial nature of these problems after cancer treatment. Sexual dysfunction can include loss of sexual desire and arousal or orgasm difficulties.[9] Survivors at the highest risk for treatment-related sexual dysfunction are those with tumors that involve the sexual or pelvic organs, following surgery or injury to autonomic nerves, treatments that affect the hormonal systems mediating sexual function in particular desire and pleasure and could also be related to side effects of multimodal treatment—CT, RT, and hematopoietic cell transplants (HCT).[9]

■ INDICATIONS FOR FERTILITY PRESERVATION IN MEN

Fertility preservation is often possible, but to preserve the full range of options, FP approaches should be discussed as early as possible, before treatment starts. The discussion can ultimately reduce distress and improve quality of life. Another discussion and/or referral may be necessary when the patient returns for follow-up and if pregnancy is being considered. The discussions should be documented in the medical record. The indications for FP in men are illustrated in **Table 1**.

TABLE 1: Indications for FP in men.

Indication	Condition
FP for cancer in men:[4]	
Exposure to radiotherapy or chemotherapy	• Damage to spermatogonial stem cells, differentiating germ cells, and Sertoli cells can result in transient or permanent azoospermia • Damage to Leydig cells is rare, but if it occurs, it results in testosterone deficiency
Effect of cancer on fertility	• Leukemia, testicular cancer (TGCT), and lymphoma affect semen parameters, even before anticancer treatments • In leukemia, the inhibin and testosterone may be low, and LH may be high
Effect of testicular tumors	• Impair fertility by disturbing spermatogenesis by destruction of surrounding tissue, local secretion of hCG and other paracrine factors, intrascrotal temperature elevation, and alterations in local blood flow • Tumor-derived vasculogenesis, in which malignant cells give rise to endothelial cells • Congenital cryptorchidism can result in development of carcinoma in situ or testicular cancer that hinders the normal transformation of neonatal gonocytes into type A spermatogonia, which are the precursors for normal spermatogenesis

Contd...

Contd...

Indication	Condition
Effect of surgery for testicular tumors	• After orchiectomy, 50% decrease in sperm concentration occurs and 10% patients become azoospermic • Retroperitoneal lymph node dissection together with radical orchiectomy can result in fertility damage due to injury of the adjacent sympathetic ganglia, which are responsible for emission and ejaculation that can result in anejaculation
FP for nononcological conditions in men:	

Exposure to gonadotoxic agent when HSCT is required	• *Hematological disorders:*
	  – Sickle cell anemia
	  – Thalassemia major
	  – Aplastic anemia
	  – Fanconi anemia
	• Primary immunodeficiencies
	• *Severe autoimmune diseases unresponsive to immunosuppressive treatment:*
	  – Juvenile and adult idiopathic arthritis
	  – SLE
	  – Systemic sclerosis
	  – Immune cytopenias
	• Osteoporosis
	• *Enzyme deficiency disease:* Hurler's syndrome

Risk of testicular degeneration	• *Chromosomal and genetic abnormalities:* – Klinefelter syndrome
Transgender– transwomen	Prior to initiation of hormonal therapy and correctable surgery

(FP: fertility preservation; hCG: human chorionic gonadotropin; HSCT: hemopoietic stem cell transplant; LH: luteinizing hormone; TGCT: testicular germ cell tumors; SLE: systemic lupus erythematosus)

Fertility preservation and method used depends on age, type of disease, spread of the disease, planned treatment, type and dose of adjuvant therapy, and time available before CT/RT. There are other issues that need to be addressed before recommending any FP modality. These are highlighted in **Box 1**.

The different FP options are depicted in **Flowchart 3**. Sperm cryopreservation is an effective and proven method of FP in males treated for cancer.[15-22] Testicular tissue or spermatogonial cryopreservation is still experimental but is the only option in prepubertal boys. Gonadal protection through hormonal manipulation is ineffective in FP in males.

BOX 1: Issues to be addressed before fertility preservation (FP).

- Oncologic prognosis and quality of life
- Availability and reliability of the FP technologies, surgical modalities, and expertise available, and costs of storage
- Fate of gametes in event of death
- Screening for hepatitis, syphilis, and human immunodeficiency virus (HIV)
- Explaining the meaning of success
- Psychosocial perspective
- Individual/parent/couple counseling
- Obtaining informed consent

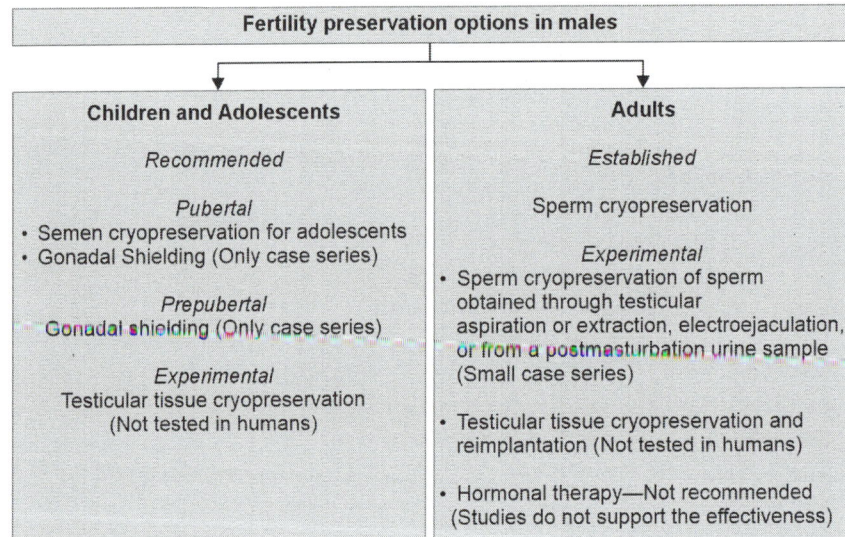

Flowchart 3: Fertility preservation techniques in the males.

Chemotherapy, radiation, or their combination results in a significant reduction of sperm quality and therefore, it is best to cryopreserve sperm before initiation of therapy.[23] The most significant factors that govern post-treatment semen quality and recovery of spermatogenesis are the age of the patient, the type of cancer, the pretreatment sperm concentrations, and the type of CT and dose of RT offered.[23]

The semen collection in adolescents and adults can be done by following methods:
- Ejaculation and semen cryopreservation
- Penile vibratory stimulation
- Electroejaculation under anesthesia
- Percutaneous epididymal sperm aspiration (PESA)—often can be performed with other procedures
- Testicular sperm aspiration (TESA)

} If ejaculation and semen collection not possible

FERTILITY PRESERVATION IN PREPUBERTAL BOYS

Isolation and cryopreservation of SSCs from the prepubertal testis before CT is possible. This technique requires a testicular biopsy and cryopreservation of either whole tissue or isolated cells. In vitro maturation of cryopreserved testicular tissue is a promising strategy for growing mature sperm for prepubertal boys. Autologous SSC transplant is an exciting technique that has demonstrated success in restoring spermatogenesis in many nonprimate models for more than 15 years and most recently, in primates.

No human studies have yet demonstrated success with in vitro maturation of sperm, a critical step toward using testicular tissue for in vitro fertilization (IVF), nor demonstrated success with testicular cell transplantation and resumption of normal spermatogenesis.[24]

ROLE OF FERTILITY-SPARING SURGERIES IN MEN

Partial orchiectomy can be done in selected patients when the testicular mass is small and radical orchiectomy may result in anorchia.[25] The German Testicular Cancer Study Group reported a 98.6% disease-free survival rate at 7-year follow-up after conservative surgery for tumors <2 cm in 73 patients.[26] However, the benefits must be weighed against the risk of tumor recurrence in these patients. In men with azoospermia undergoing orchidectomy, sperms can be extracted from the epididymis and vas deferens of the orchiectomy specimen. Sperm may also be recovered from the contralateral noncancerous testicle at the time of orchiectomy in patients with azoospermia.[27] These sperms retrieved can be cryopreserved to preserve fertility.[28,14] Sperm banking before surgery, even in patients undergoing partial orchiectomy, is advisable. Oncologic surgery for prostate, bladder, or colon cancer may damage nerves and affect potency or ejaculation; thus, careful dissection during these surgeries to prevent nerve damage is necessary.

REASONS FOR NOT OFFERING FERTILITY PRESERVATION

Young men with cancer experience low referral rates for fertility counseling and sperm banking. This may be related to lack of communication, limited resources and time, perceived high cost, physician and patient modesty, provider knowledge gaps, and urgency to begin treatment.[29]

RECOVERY OF HUMAN SPERMATOGENESIS AFTER CANCER THERAPY

The survival and ability of mitotically quiescent spermatogonia to resume mitotic activity and to produce differentiating spermatogonia affect spermatogenesis recovery after a cytotoxic treatment is variable.

Recolonization of surviving spermatogonia can first be detected 6 months after a dose of 0.2 Gy, 9–18 months after a dose of 1 Gy, and >4 years after a dose of 10 Gy.[9,30] Complete destruction of SSCs after RT is some patients is thought to be the main cause of permanent infertility.

Men treated with alkylating agents such as cyclophosphamide had lower sperm retrieval rates, ranging from 26 to 36%.[9,30] After high-dose cyclophosphamide treatment, sperms were seen in the ejaculate after a recovery period of 1 year and cyclophosphamide combined with busulfan or thiotepa presented initial sperm recovery after 3 years.[30] Men who received platinum drugs (those treated for testicular cancer) had the highest rate of sperm retrieval at 85%. Overall presence of sperms was seen in 37% of male cancer survivors and in 42.9% of individual procedures.[30] Subsequent ICSI resulted in slightly more than 57% fertilization rate and a pregnancy rate of 50%.[30]

SAFETY OF CHILDREN BORN AFTER CANCER TREATMENT OF FATHER

The reports on the health of the offspring of male cancer survivors are conflicting. Some studies show a small increase in the risk of anomalies and cancers in children. Childhood cancer survivors seem to be more at risk than young adult survivors. The risk seems to be higher in the period immediately after cancer therapy. Cancer patients seem to have higher incidences of genetic aberrations than the general population. Avoiding childbearing immediately after cancer therapy seems to be prudent as recommended by the European Society for Medical Oncology (12 months).[31] The potential harm to sperm deoxyribonucleic acid (DNA) integrity from cancer therapies, especially in the era of assisted reproductive technology (ART) which has allowed the use of sperm that would not otherwise be capable of naturally fertilizing an oocyte, has led to concern about the health of the offspring of cancer survivors.[32] Pretreatment sperm cryopreservation can circumvent the effects of cancer therapies. Further surveillance of the children is required, especially those born after ART. Further studies are required to look into the molecular biological mechanism involved in different cancers. Overall data on the health of children born to cancer survivor fathers is encouraging with no increased risk of congenital abnormalities, genetic disease, and abnormal karyotype.[33]

ETHICAL ISSUES

In case of demise, cryopreserved tissue and sperms should be treated as per the instructions in the consent or advance directive or any other reliable indicator of consent.[34] If consented to, it can be used for the treatment of the partner (consent form from surviving spouse or partner needed). Parents cannot utilize cryopreserved tissue or sperms unless prior legal rights have been given to them by the affected individual. Even if not consented for use in a partner, consideration can be given upon such a request coming after a period of grieving. Posthumous extraction can be requested by a partner or spouse but not by parents but requires legal permission.[35]

CONCLUSION

Preserving the reproductive function is necessary and the future of those in need requires increased patient awareness and understanding. This can occur only with the integration of FP services with oncological services and other specialties such as immunologists, hematologists, and surgeons. Patient navigation by social workers facilitates patients in taking efficient care and coordination with both the treating physician and reproductive care specialist. Key recommendations for oncofertility care pathway risk communication, referral to a fertility specialist, and counseling followed by decision making. By talking to patients about their options to preserve fertility at the earliest phase of the treatment plan provides a positive prognosis for the outcome and reinforces the positive message of hope. There is a need to develop a stronger partnership between the fields of oncology and reproductive medicine to improve access to FP services for oncology patients. Such processes would ensure the optimization of services so that all cancer patients would receive the best care in protecting their fertility.

REFERENCES

1. Schover LR, Brey K, Lichtin A, Lipshultz LI, Jeha S. Oncologists' attitudes and practices regarding banking sperm before cancer treatment. J Clin Oncol. 2002;20:1890-7.
2. Achille MA, Rosberger Z, Robitaille R, Lebel S, Gouin JP, Bultz BD, et al. Facilitators and obstacles to sperm banking in young men receiving gonadotoxic chemotherapy for cancer: The perspective of survivors and health care professionals. Hum Reprod. 2006;21:3206-16.
3. Hotaling JM, Lopushnyan NA, Davenport M, Christensen H, Pagel ER, Muller CH, et al. Raw and test-thaw semen parameters after cryopreservation among men with newly diagnosed cancer. Fertil Steril. 2013;99(2):464-9.
4. Michailov Y, Lunenfeld E, Kapelushnik J, Huleihel M. Leukemia and male infertility: past, present, and future. Leuk Lymphoma. 2019;60(5):1126-35.
5. Martinez G, Walschaerts M, Le Mitouard M, Borye R, Thomas C, Auger J, et al. Impact of Hodgkin or non-Hodgkin lymphoma and their treatments on sperm aneuploidy: a prospective study by the French CECOS network. Fertil Steril. 2017;107(2):341-50.
6. Rives N, Perdrix A, Hennebicq S, Saïas-Magnan J, Melin MC, Berthaut I, et al. The semen quality of 1158 men with testicular cancer at the time of cryopreservation: results of the French National CECOS Network. J Androl. 2012;33(6):1394-401.

7. Vakalopoulos I, Dimou P, Anagnostou I, Zeginiadou T. Impact of cancer and cancer treatment on male fertility. Hormones. 2015;14(4):579-89.
8. Himpe J, Lammerant S, Van den Bergh L, Lapeire L, De Roo C. The impact of systemic oncological treatments on the fertility of adolescents and young adults: a systematic review. Life. 2023;13(5):1209.
9. Howell SJ, Shalet SM. Spermatogenesis after cancer treatment: damage and recovery. J Natl Cancer Inst Monogr. 2005;34:12-7.
10. Ceccarelli C, Canale D, Vitti P. Radioactive iodine (^{131}I) effects on male fertility. Curr Opin Urol. 2008;18(6):598-601.
11. Albers P, Albrecht W, Algaba F, Bokemeyer C, Cohn-Cedermark G, Horwich A, et al. Guidelines on Testicular Cancer: 2015 Update. Eur Urol. 2015;68(6):1054-68.
12. Petersen PM, Giwercman A, Daugaard G, Rørth M, Petersen JH, Skakkeaek NE, et al. Effect of graded testicular doses of radiotherapy in patients treated for carcinoma-in-situ in the testis. J Clin Oncol. 2002;20(6):1537-43.
13. Yaish I, Azem F, Gutfeld O, Silman Z, Serebro M, Sharon O, et al. A single radioactive iodine treatment has a deleterious effect on ovarian reserve in women with thyroid cancer: results of a prospective pilot study. Thyroid. 2018; 28(4):522-7.
14. Choi BB, Goldstein M, Moomjy M, Palermo G, Rosenwaks Z, Schlegel PN. Births using sperm retrieved via immediate microdissection of a solitary testis with cancer. Fertil Steril. 2005;84(5):1508-e1.
15. Hourvitz A, Goldschlag DE, Davis OK, Gosden LV, Palermo GD, Rosenwaks Z. Intracytoplasmic sperm injection (ICSI) using cryopreserved sperm from men with malignant neoplasm yields high pregnancy rates. Fertil Steril. 2008;90:557-63.
16. Romerius P, Ståhl O, Moëll C, Relander T, Cavallin-Ståhl E, Gustafsson H, et al. Sperm DNA integrity in men treated for childhood cancer. Clin Cancer Res. 2010;16:3843-50.
17. Salonia A, Gallina A, Matloob R, Rocchini L, Saccà A, Abdollah F, et al. Is sperm banking of interest to patients with nongerm cell urological cancer before potentially fertility damaging treatments? J Urol. 2009;182:1101-7.
18. Schmidt KT, Andersen CY. Recommendations for fertility preservation in patients with lymphomas. J Assist Reprod Genet. 2012;29:473-7.
19. Chang HC, Chen SC, Chen J, Hsieh JT. Initial 10-year experience of sperm cryopreservation services for cancer patients. J Formos Med Assoc. 2006;105(12): 1022-6.
20. Yee S, Fuller-Thomson E, Dwyer C, Greenblatt E, Shapiro H. Just what the doctor ordered: Factors associated with oncology patients' decision to bank sperm. Can Urol Assoc J. 2012;6:E174-8.
21. Ping P, Zhu WB, Zhang XZ, Yao KS, Xu P, Huang YR, et al. Sperm banking for male reproductive preservation: a 6-year retrospective multi-centre study in China. Asian J Androl. 2010;12(3):356.
22. Navarro Medina P, Barroso Deyne E, Castillo Suárez M, Blanco Diez A, Lozano M, Artiles Hernández JL, et al. An analysis of our experience in cryopreservation of semen from cancer patients [in Spanish]. Actas Urol Esp. 2010;34:101-5.
23. Trottmann M, Becker AJ, Stadler T, Straub J, Soljanik I, Schlenker B, et al. Semen quality in men with malignant diseases before and after therapy and the role of cryopreservation. Eur Urol. 2007;52(2):355-67.

24. Goossens E, Jahnukainen K, Mitchell RT, Van Pelt AM, Pennings G, Rives N, et al. Fertility preservation in boys: recent developments and new insights. Hum Reprod Open. 2020;2020(3):hoaa016.
25. Sabanegh ES Jr, Ragheb AM. Male fertility after cancer. Urology. 2009;73(2):225-31.
26. Heidenreich A, Weissbach L, Höltl W, Albers P, Kliesch S, Köhrmann KU, et al. Organ sparing surgery for malignant germ cell tumor of the testis. J Urol. 2001;166(6):2161-5.
27. Schrader M, Müller M, Sofikitis N, Straub B, Krause H, Miller K. Oncotese: testicular sperm extraction in azoospermic cancer patients before chemotherapy-new guidelines? Urology. 2003;61(2):421-5.
28. Baniel J, Sella A. Sperm extraction at orchiectomy for testis cancer. Fertil Steril. 2001;75(2):260-2.
29. Grover NS, Deal AM, Wood WA, Mersereau JE. Young men with cancer experience low referral rates for fertility counseling and sperm banking. J Oncol Pract. 2016;12(5):465-71.
30. Okada K, Fujisawa M. Recovery of spermatogenesis following cancer treatment with cytotoxic chemotherapy and radiotherapy. World J Mens Health. 2019;37(2):166.
31. Peccatori FA, Azim HA, Orecchia R, Hoekstra HJ, Pavlidis N, Kesic V, et al. Cancer, pregnancy and fertility: ESMO Clinical Practice Guidelines for diagnosis, treatment and follow-up. Ann Oncol. 2013;24:vi160-70.
32. Winther JF, Boice JD, Mulvihill JJ, Stovall M, Frederiksen K, Tawn EJ, et al. Chromosomal abnormalities among offspring of childhood-cancer survivors in Denmark: a population-based study. Am J Hum Genet. 2004;74(6):1282-5.
33. Delessard M, Saulnier J, Rives A, Dumont L, Rondanino C, Rives N. Exposure to chemotherapy during childhood or adulthood and consequences on spermatogenesis and male fertility. Int J Mol Sci. 2020;21(4):1454.
34. Grin L, Girsh E, Harlev A. Male fertility preservation: methods, indications and challenges. Andrologia. 2021;53(2):e13635.
35. Sharma AP, Kaur J, Mavuduru RS, Bora GS, Devana SK, Singh SK, et al. Fertility preservation in men: Perspective. Indian J Urol. 2018;34(4):241-4.

Index

Page numbers followed by *f* refer to figure, *fc* refer to flowchart, and *t* refer to table

A

Acrosomal reaction 17
Alcohol intake 9
Alkaline 13
  seminal vesicular fluid 13
American Society for Reproductive Medicine 9
American Society of Clinical Oncology guidelines 54
Anabolic-androgenic steroids 10
Anejaculation 15
Anemia, aplastic 57
Anesthesia 58
Antioxidants 44
Antisperm antibody 5, 17
Arthritis, idiopathic 57
Artificial intelligence 41
Ascorbic acid 47
Aspermia 17
Assisted reproductive technique 1, 3, 15, 20, 29, , 33, 49, 60
Asthenozoospermia 15, 17
Autoimmune diseases, severe 57
Azoospermia 7, 8, 18, 30, 33, 33
  nonobstructive 6, 21, 28, 37
  type of 40
Azoospermic male, evaluation of 6*fc*, 28

B

Biomaterials 41
Body mass index 8
Buffalo hump 16

C

Cancer, effects of 56
Capacitation 17
Carnitines 46
Cavernosal artery 24*f*
Central hypothalamo-pituitary forms 5
Chemiluminescence test 18
Chemotherapeutic agents 55*fc*
Chemotherapy 5, 54, 56, 58
Chromosomal abnormalities 41, 57
Coenzyme Q10 44, 46
  chemical structure of 46*f*
Computed tomography scan 20, 25
Core tissue extraction 38*f*
Cowper's glands 13
Cranial irradiation 55
  effects of 55
Cushing's disease 16
Cystic fibrosis transmembrane conductance regulator 3, 6, 16
Cytotoxic agents 54*fc*

D

Deoxyribonucleic acid 8, 17, 44, 44*f*, 60
  fragmentation index 9, 17
  integrity test 17
Diet 11
Dietary supplements 43
Docosahexaenoic acid 50
Doppler
  sonography 24*f*
  study 23
  ultrasound 21

E

Eicosapentaenoic acid 50
Ejaculate, absence of 13
Ejaculation 58
Ejaculatory duct 22
  obstruction 14, 30
Ejaculatory failure 39
Electroejaculation 58
End-diastolic velocity 23
Endocrine system 54
Endocrinopathy 15
Enzyme deficiency disease 57
Eosin staining 17

Eosin-nigrosin staining 17
Epididymal ductules 21
Epididymal isolated cysts 22
Epididymis 33
Estradiol 4, 8
    levels 16, 40
European Association of Urology 13

F

Fanconi anemia 57
Fatty acids 50
Fertility 22, 55, 56
    preservation 53, 56-59
        indications for 56
        techniques 58*fc*
    sparing surgeries, role of 59
Fine needle
    aspiration 28
    biopsy 28
Folic acid 48
Follicle-stimulating
    hormone 3-6, 16, 28, 40, 46

G

Gamete donation 41
Genetic
    counseling 41
    evaluation 18
    factors 39, 41
    screening 4
    testing 18, 41
Germ cell 54
Glutathione 50
    chemical structure of 50
    supplementation 50
Gonadotoxicity, mechanisms of 55
Gonadotropin-releasing
    hormone agonists 39
Gynecomastia 3, 15

H

Hair distribution 15
Hematological disorders 57
Hematopoietic cell transplants 56, 57
Hormonal stimulation 39
Hormonal therapy 39, 57
Human chorionic gonadotropin 39, 57
Human spermatogenesis after cancer
    therapy, recovery of 59

Hurler's syndrome 57
Hybrid techniques 37
Hydrocele, presence of 16
Hydrogen peroxide 18
Hydroxyl radicals 18
Hypergonadotropic hypogonadism 16
Hyperinsulinemia 8
Hyperprolactinemia 16
Hypogonadism 3
    anabolic steroid-induced 10
    secondary 5, 16
Hypogonadotropic hypogonadism 5
Hypo-osmotic swelling test 17
Hypoplasia 23
Hypospadias 3
Hypothalamic-pituitary-adrenal axis 10
    endocrinological abnormality of 8

I

Immotility 2
Immune cytopenia 57
Immunobead test 17
Impaired sperm function 44*f*
In vitro fertilization 28, 47, 59
Inferior vena cava 25
Infertile couple 13
    initial evaluation of 3*fc*
Infertility 1, 10, 20, 28
Intracytoplasmic sperm
    injection 15, 28, 33
Intrauterine insemination 15, 21

K

Karyotyping 5
Klinefelter syndrome 37, 57

L

L-arginine 48
    chemical structure of 49*f*
L-carnitine, chemical structure of 46*f*
Leukemia 54, 56
Leukocytes 2, 14, 15
Leukospermia 15
Leydig cell 10
    damage 5
    injury 54
Low-level radiofrequency electromagnetic
    field 10
Luteinizing hormone 4, 5, 16, 40, 54, 57

Index

Lycopene 47
  chemical structure of 47f
  supplementation 47

M

Machine learning 41
Macroadenomas 24
Magnetic resonance imaging 20, 24, 25f
Male hormonal assay 5t
Male infertility 8, 20, 21, 23, 26, 41, 43, 44f
  evaluation of 1, 20
  surgical management of 28
Male reproductive health 43
Melatonin, chemical structure of 49
Mesenchymal stem cells 41
Microadenomas 24
Microscopic epididymal sperm
  aspiration 31, 33
Microtesticular sperm extraction 30
Mitochondrial membrane potential 8
Mixed antiglobulin reaction test 17
Mobile phones, effects of 10
Moon face 16

N

N-acetyl cysteine 49
  chemical structure of 49f
Nanotechnology 41
Necrozoospermia 39
Needle
  aspiration biopsy 35
  testicular sperm extraction 35
Neutralize reactive oxygen species 44
Nitric oxide 18, 48
Nitroblue tetrazolium test 18
Nonprogressive motility 2, 14
Normal hormonal screening tests 7
Nutraceuticals 43
Nutrition 43

O

Obesity 8
Obstructive azoospermia 6, 16, 21, 30, 40
Oligoasthenozoospermia 51
Oligospermia 8
Oligozoospermia 16, 51
  severe 18
Omega-3 fatty acids 50
Oncofertility 53

Open fine needle aspiration 34
Open testicular biopsy 28
Optimizing sperm retrieval strategies 39
Orchiectomy 57
Osteoporosis 57

P

Peak systolic velocity 23
Penile vibratory stimulation 58
Penis, examination of 3, 16
Percutaneous epididymal
  sperm aspiration 30, 34, 58
  procedure 34f
  sample 35f
Peyronie plaques 3
Pharmaceuticals 43
Phimosis 3
Poor sperm motility 43
Postcoital test 17
Postejaculatory urine analysis 15
Post-testicular absence 5
Pregnancy losses, recurrent 2
Preimplantation genetic testing 41
Pretreatment sperm cryopreservation 60
Progressive motility 2, 14
Prolactin 4, 16
Prostaglandin E1 23
Prostate evaluation 22
Prostatic secretion 13
Prostatic urethra cysts 24
Pyospermia 15

R

Radiation 58
Radioactive iodine
  dose of 55
  effects of 55
Radiotherapy 54, 56
  effects of 55
Reactive oxygen species 17, 44f
Renal cell carcinoma 4
Reproductive rights 42
Retrieve sperm 30
Retrograde ejaculation 5, 13

S

Scrotal ultrasound 7, 17, 21
Scrotum 25f

Selective androgen receptor
　　modulators 41
Selenium 48
Semen
　　analysis 2t, 4, 5, 13, 14t
　　　　parameters, abnormal 15
　　collection 58
　　concentration 2
　　cryopreservation 58
　　investigations 13
　　pH of 13
　　quality 9, 10
　　specimen 13
　　volume 2, 13, 17, 14, 17
Seminal fructose 14
Seminal vesicles 22
　　transrectal ultrasound image of 23f
Seminal vesicular secretion 13
Sertoli only syndrome 37f
Sexual characteristics, secondary 3
Sexual dysfunction 56
Sickle cell anemia 57
Single seminiferous tubule 37
Skin 15
Sperm
　　agglutination 17
　　cells 48
　　concentration 14
　　delivery 29
　　deoxyribonucleic acid 5
　　　　fragmentation 17
　　function tests 13, 17
　　morphology 15
　　　　abnormal 43
　　　　assessment of 15
　　motility 15
　　penetration assays 17
　　production 29
　　retrieval 37, 39, 40
　　　　efficacy of 39
　　　　techniques for 33, 35
　　selection of 15
　　vitality tests 14, 17
Spermatogenesis 5, 9, 10, 28
　　follicle-stimulating hormone 54
Spermatogenic failure, primary 5, 16
Spermatogonial stem cell 41, 54, 55
Spermatozoa 14, 30
Spermicidal lubricants 13

Stem cell therapy 41
Stress 10
Successful sperm retrieval, predictors of 40
Superoxide anions 18
Surgery 30, 54
　　effects of 57
Systemic lupus erythematosus 57
Systemic sclerosis 57

T

Teratospermia 15
Testicular
　　atrophy 10, 22
　　biopsy 7, 40
　　cancer 56
　　degeneration, risk of 57
　　fine needle aspiration biopsy 35
　　forms, primary 5
　　germ cell tumors 57
　　histology 39, 40
　　mapping 28
　　size 5, 15
　　sperm
　　　　aspiration 30, 35, 35f, 58
　　　　extraction 30
　　tumors 57
　　　　effects of 56
　　　　primary 22
　　volume, enlarged 21
Testis 35, 25f
　　normal 22f
　　small 22f
　　undescended 24
Testosterone 4, 5, 10, 16, 40, 54
Thalassemia major 57
Thyroid-stimulating hormone 4, 16
Total motile sperm count 14
Total sperm count 14
Toxicity, degree of 54
Traditional semen analysis 20
Transabdominal ultrasound 22
Transrectal ultrasound scan 21
Tyrosine kinase inhibitors 54

U

Ultrasound 21
　　guided techniques 40

V

Valsalva maneuver 24
Varicocele 3, 16, 23, 24, 29
   presence of 16
Vas
   bilateral absence of 16
   deferens 22
      absence of 14
      congenital absence of 18, 21
      terminal 22
   obstruction of 5
Vascular assessment 21
Vasectomy 29
Vasography 20, 25
Venography 20, 25
Vitamin 44
   B9 48
   C 44, 47, 50
   D 47, 48
      deficiency 48
      localization of 48
   E 44, 47, 50
      supplementation 47

W

World Health Organization 11, 13

Y

Y-chromosome microdeletions 41

Z

Zinc 48